Praise for *Eat Move Sleep*

"A passionate and practical guide to living better and longer. *Eat Move Sleep* will change your life. It might also save it."

—**SIR KEN ROBINSON, Ph.D.**,
author of *The Element* and *Finding Your Element*

"One of the most successful nonfiction writers of his generation, Tom Rath has produced a blockbuster book with deep insights alongside specific actions. *Eat Move Sleep* is a transformative work."

—**DANIEL H. PINK**, author of *Drive* and *To Sell Is Human*

"Tom Rath lays out ways of changing our eating, exercise, and sleeping habits that are easy to do at our own pace. *Eat Move Sleep* will be a big help to me and my patients."

—**GORDY KLATT, M.D.**, founder of the
American Cancer Society Relay for Life

"You can't stop reading ... your health IQ will never be the same."

—**PATRICK LENCIONI**, author of
The Five Dysfunctions of a Team and *The Advantage*

"Tom Rath has developed multiple creative strategies for a lifestyle of enduring health.

—**CALDWELL B ESSELSTYN, JR., M.D.**,
author of *Prevent and Reverse Heart Disease*

"Rath's new book invaluably delivers."

—**BRIAN WANSINK, Ph.D.**,
author of *Mindless Eating* and *Slim by Design*

"Backed by science and filled with heart, *Eat Move Sleep* is the best self-improvement book I've ever read."

—**ORI BRAFMAN**, author of *Sway* and *The Chaos Imperative*

"*Eat Move Sleep* never lets the reader off the hook. All 76 million of us baby boomers should take heed."

—**MERYL COMER**, President,
Geoffrey Beene Foundation, Alzheimer's Initiative

"The new operating code for human health. Reading *Eat Move Sleep* should be as mandatory as health insurance."

—**SHAWN ACHOR**, author of
The Happiness Advantage and *Before Happiness*

"As a physician, I cannot begin to explain how vital this book is for improving human health and well-being."

—**JASON POWERS, M.D.**, Chief Medical Officer, Right Step

"I learned surprising health secrets from Tom's lifelong research. Read *Eat Move Sleep*; you will be stronger and live longer."

—**GREG LINK**, co-founder, Covey Leadership Center

"A road map for leading a long and meaningful life. Every human being should have this book right next to the Bible on their nightstand."

—**VAL J. HALAMANDARIS**, President,
National Association for Homecare and Hospice

"Tom Rath knows this topic inside out and is sharing his best research-driven tips and proven ideas."

—**KEN BLANCHARD, Ph.D.**, coauthor of
The One Minute Manager and *Fit at Last*

"Being healthy begins by reading this life-changing book."

—**ANITA BRUZZESE**, author, *USA Today* columnist

"Filled with valuable tips, this book will help you evaluate and improve your health by making simple changes."

—**CRAIG GROESCHEL**, Senior Pastor of LifeChurch.tv

EAT MOVE SLEEP

How Small Choices Lead to Big Changes

TOM RATH

MISSIONDAY

Library of Congress Control Number: 2013935905
ISBN: 978-1-939714-00-8 (hardcover)
ISBN: 978-1-939714-01-5 (digital edition)
ISBN: 978-1-939714-02-2 (international edition)
First Printing: 2013
10 9 8 7 6 5 4 3 2 1

Bulk purchase discounts, special editions, and customized excerpts are available direct from the publisher. For information about books for educational, business, or promotional purposes, please email: SPmarkets@missionday.com
Submit all other publisher requests to inquires@missionday.com

To book this author for a speaking engagement, contact the Missionday Speakers Bureau: speaking@missionday.com

Author's website: **www.tomrath.org**

To my wife Ashley, daughter Harper, and son Everett who brighten each day ... and make the prospect of tomorrow even better

CONTENTS

CONTENTS

EAT MOVE SLEEP

Eat Move Sleep

Choices count. You can make decisions today that will give you more energy tomorrow. The right choices over time greatly improve your odds of a long and healthy life.

A hundred years ago, many people died from infectious diseases because they had no cure. But today, a majority of people die from preventable conditions. The next time you are with two friends, consider that two of the three of you are likely to die from heart disease or cancer.

The problem is, you do not see the threats that your small daily decisions pose in the moment. You have little urgency to change your diet until all those years of fried food, sugar, and processed meat cause a heart attack at age 60. At that point, reversing disease is possible but more difficult.

No matter how healthy you are today, you can take specific actions to have more energy and live longer. Regardless of your age, you can make better choices in the moment. Small decisions — about how you eat, move, and sleep each day — count more than you think. As I have learned from personal experience, these choices shape your life.

A Personal Perspective

At age 16, I was playing basketball with friends when I noticed something wrong with my vision. There was a black circle in the middle of my visual field. I assumed it would go away. Instead, it got progressively worse. I finally told my mom, who immediately took me to an eye doctor.

That black spot turned out to be a large tumor on the back of my left eye. The doctor said it might lead to blindness. As if that was not enough, I needed to get a blood test to rule out other medical problems. A few weeks later, my mom and I went back to the doctor's office for the results.

The doctor told us I had a rare genetic disorder called Von Hippel-Lindau (VHL). While VHL typically runs in families, my condition was a new mutation that affects just one in every 4,400,000 people. This mutation essentially shuts off a powerful tumor suppressor gene and leads to rampant cancerous growth throughout the body.

I still vividly recall sitting on one side of a large wooden desk as my doctor tried to explain what it would be like to battle cancer for the rest of my life. It was one of those moments when your stomach sinks and your mind races for an alternate explanation. My doctor then described how I was also likely to develop cancer in my kidneys, adrenal glands, pancreas, brain, and spine.

While the thought of losing my eyesight was tough, these longer-term issues were even more daunting. That conversation with the doctor forced me to wrestle with much larger questions about my life. Would people treat me differently if they knew about my illness? Was there any chance I would get married and have kids? Perhaps most importantly, I wondered if there was any way I could live a long and healthy life.

Doctors tried everything to save my eyesight, from freezing the tumors to cooking them with a laser. But the sight in my eye never returned. Once I got over this loss, I turned my attention to learning everything I could about the other manifestations of this rare disease.

I quickly realized that the more I learned, the more I could do to increase my odds of living longer. As new information emerged, I discovered I could stay ahead of my condition with annual MRIs, CTs, and eye exams. If doctors caught tumors early when they were small, the tumors were less likely to spread and kill me. Learning that was a huge relief. Even if it required some difficult surgeries, there was something I could do to live longer.

I have had annual exams and scans for 20 years now and currently have small tumors in my kidneys, adrenal glands, pancreas, spine, and brain. Every year, I "watch and wait" to find out if any of these tumors are large enough to require surgery. In most cases, they are not.

Waiting around for active tumors to grow may sound nerve-wracking. It could be, if I dwelled on the genetic condition that is beyond my control. Instead, I use these annual exams to stay focused on what I can do to decrease the odds of my cancers growing and spreading.

As each year goes by, I learn more about how I can eat, move, and sleep to improve my chances of living a long and healthy life. Then I apply what I learn to make better choices. I act as if my life depends on each decision. Because it does.

Small Choices Change Everything

Making better choices takes work. There is a daily give and take, but it is worth the effort. The vast knowledge we have to prevent cancer, heart disease, and other chronic illnesses is staggering. Every day, I read about new ideas that could help someone I care about live a longer and healthier life.

Over the last decade, I have dedicated a great deal of time to organizing this virtual sea of information in a way that can benefit others. What I look for are simple and proven ideas. I read a wide range of academic studies and research-based articles — from medical and psychological journals to in-depth books — and try to extract knowledge that can help people make better decisions and live healthier lives.

Let me be clear. I am not a doctor. Nor am I an expert on nutrition, exercise physiology, or sleep disorders. I am just a patient. I also happen to be a researcher and voracious reader who loves to extract valuable findings and share them with friends. In this book, you will find the most credible and practical ideas I have found so far.

What I learned from all this research influences my countless daily decisions. Every bite of food either increases or decreases my odds of spending a few more years with my wife and two young children. Half an hour of exercise in the morning makes for better interactions all day. Then a sound night of sleep gives me energy to tackle the next day. I am a more active parent, a better spouse, and more engaged in my work when I eat, move, and sleep well.

What seem like small or inconsequential moments accumulate rapidly. When your good daily decisions outweigh your poor ones, you boost your chances of growing old in better health. Life itself is a big game of beating the odds. Take, for example, these four largely preventable diseases: cancer, diabetes, heart disease, and lung disease. Combined, they kill nearly 9 in 10 people.

Researchers have estimated that 90 percent of us could live to age 90 with some simple lifestyle choices. What's more, we could live free of common diseases that make our final years miserable. Even if you have a family history of heart disease or cancer, most of your fate is in your control.

A recent study suggests you do not "inherit" longevity as much as previously believed. Instead, the sum of your habits determines your life span. How long you live is more about how you live your life and less about how long your parents lived.

I am a living testament to the fact that lousy predispositions can be encoded in your genes. Yet even in this extreme case, my decisions affect the odds of new tumors growing and my existing cancers spreading. The reality is, the majority of your risk in life lies in the choices you make, not in your family tree.

No single act can prevent cancer or guarantee you will live a long life. Anyone who promises you something that absolute is a fraud. What I will share in this book are some of the most practical ideas to improve your odds of a longer, healthier, and more fulfilling life.

30 Days to Better Decisions

As you read this book, I hope you find ideas that work for you and test them over the next month. From my own experience and from observing others, I have noticed that making better choices often becomes automatic after just a couple of weeks. However, it takes some initiative — on your own, with a friend, or as part of a group — to take the first step.

Each chapter has three research-based findings and concludes with three ideas for how you can apply them in your life. Challenge yourself to use at least one idea per day for the next month. Write them down. Post them somewhere in your home or office. See if you can make good decisions automatic.

If one of these strategies works for you, stick with it. If not, move on to the next one. It's up to you to determine which ideas make sense and can improve your life the most. No one can do everything in this book, period. But you should be able to add at least a few ideas into your daily routine. On the book's website at www.eatmovesleep.org, you can:

- Create a personalized *Eat Move Sleep Plan* based on your needs and behaviors
- Use the *Reference Explorer* for direct links to more than 400 academic journals, books, articles, and notes
- Download the *First 30 Days Challenge* and other tools to use with friends, groups, and teams

Have fun. The key is to create a plan that works for your unique situation. If you apply some of the ideas with at least one friend, you can greatly increase your odds of building new habits. Or, if you prefer to test things as you go, keep moving at your own pace. Creating a few new patterns in the next month will lead to healthier choices for years to come.

The Eat, Move, Sleep Equation

Starting your day with a healthy breakfast increases your odds of being active in the hours that follow. This helps you eat well throughout the day. Consuming the right foods and adding activity makes for a much better night's sleep. This sound night of sleep will make it even easier to eat well and move more tomorrow.

In contrast, a lousy night of sleep immediately threatens the other two areas. That bad night of sleep makes you crave a less healthy breakfast and decreases your odds of being active. In the worst-case scenario, all three elements start to work against you, creating a downward spiral that makes each day progressively worse. This is why the book is structured to help you work on *all three elements together*.

New research shows that tackling multiple elements *at the same time* increases your odds of success, compared to initiating a new diet or exercise program in isolation. Eating, moving, and sleeping well are even *easier* if you work on all three simultaneously. These three ingredients for a good day build on one another. When these elements are working together, they create an upward spiral and progressively better days.

If you eat, move, and sleep well today, you will have more energy tomorrow. You will treat your friends and family better. You will achieve more at work and give more to your community.

It all starts with making decisions like *tomorrow* depends on it.

The Basics

Forget Fad Diets, Forever

If you find yourself confused by the latest diet trends and information, you are not alone. According to one report, three out of every four people claim that today's ever-changing dietary guidelines make it hard to eat healthy. More than half of people surveyed find it *easier to figure out their income taxes* than to know how to eat right.

This could explain why a majority of Americans are trying to lose weight, yet two-thirds are overweight or obese. One problem is that being "on a diet" is a temporary effort that assumes an endpoint. Many popular diets are destined to fail. When you see a book or advertisement claiming you can be healthy by doing just one thing for weeks on end, stop and think about the ramifications.

If your primary goal is weight loss, there are countless fad diets to temporarily shed pounds, yet they do not serve your long-term interests. Some of the most egregious examples are diets that instruct you to eat only cookies (yes, several of these exist) or drink smoothies for several days. Even if you do shed a few pounds in the short term, this works *against* your overall health.

Even mainstream diets fail if they target a single element at the expense of the whole equation. In the early 1990s, "low fat" was the most popular type of diet. This led food companies to create products with lower overall fat. Bagel shops began to appear on every corner. Low-fat chips and crackers lined grocery store aisles. I was one of many who consumed about anything with low fat content, in hopes of being healthier.

However, this dietary shift ignored the fact that it is relatively easy to reduce total fat content by adding carbohydrates, sugars, and synthetic substitutes. This allowed food companies to replace the flavor from fatty foods with something even sweeter. To a large degree, food producers simply exchanged fats for sugar-based ingredients.

Attention then shifted to low-carb diets. This led people to consume greater amounts of animal products for protein, ignoring the detrimental impact animal fats have on our health. And, while vegetarian diets have been popular for decades, they are less healthy if animal products are replaced by refined carbs and sweet foods.

Even basic calorie counting is insufficient. As one expert put it, "Contrary to nutritional dogma, calories are not created equal." It turns out, the belief that you can eat *anything* in moderation is dead wrong.

The *quality* of what you eat matters far more than the overall *quantity*. This is the primary finding from a landmark Harvard study that tracked more than 100,000 people for two decades. The researchers discovered that the *types of foods* you consume influence your health more than your total caloric intake. Quality of food matters even more than levels of physical activity. As one of the Harvard researchers put it, "The notion that it's O.K. to eat everything in moderation is just an excuse to eat whatever you want."

Many popular diets have some helpful elements, but *only* if they are part of a more holistic approach to eating. Think of all the diets you have tried. Keep the best elements of these diets in mind as you make choices. For your overall approach to eating, find foods with less fat, fewer carbohydrates, and as little added sugar as possible.

Eating well does not need to be difficult or complicated. It is possible for healthy eating to be sustainable and even enjoyable. Set your sights on foods that are good for your near-term energy *and* long-term health. Making a commitment to eating the right foods every day is a lot easier than jumping from one diet to the next.

Once you start eating better, give it time — a lot of time. People often bounce from diet to diet because they grow impatient. The body takes a long time to react to these dietary changes, usually a year or more, according to experts. Instead of worrying about losing 10 pounds in the next month, focus on better decisions the next time you eat. When you make better choices in the moment, it benefits your overall health *and* well-being.

● ● ●

Make Inactivity Your Enemy

Exercise alone is not enough. Working out three times a week is not enough. Being active *throughout the day* is what keeps you healthy.

For centuries, our ancestors spent a large portion of their time moving around on foot. From the days of hunting wild animals to more recent times working on farms, a typical workday used to be spent doing physical labor. Over the past century, this has changed dramatically.

On average, we now spend more time sitting down (9.3 hours) than sleeping in a given day. The human body is not built for this, and the obesity and diabetes it contributes to is a major public health problem. Watching your diet and exercising 30 minutes a day will not be enough to offset many hours of sitting.

When I was growing up, my days were filled with physical activity. I spent most of my time running around the neighborhood with friends, playing basketball in my driveway, and practicing for other sports. When I look back, it is no wonder I felt so good and had boundless energy. Most of my waking hours were spent in motion.

This is why it was a rude awakening when I started working full time. All of a sudden, the majority of my time was spent sitting. On my best days, I would spend an hour working out. Then I spent about an hour walking around my home and office. Add eight hours of sleep, and that left about 14 hours a day of sitting in a chair, car, or couch. Not exactly the active lifestyle I was used to before signing on to a desk job.

Reducing this chronic *inactivity* is even more essential than brief periods of vigorous exercise. When scientists from the National Institutes of Health followed 240,000 adults for a decade, they discovered that exercise alone is insufficient. Even seven hours a week of moderate to vigorous physical activity was not enough to keep people alive. Among the most active group studied, who exercised more than seven hours a week, those who spent the most time sitting had a 50 percent greater risk of death from any cause. They also *doubled* their odds of dying from heart disease. Exercise clearly helps, but it will not offset several hours of sitting.

The amount of time you spend seated adds up quickly. Let's do the math. You might sit down for a while to watch the morning news and eat breakfast. Then let's say your commute adds another 30 to 60 minutes sitting in a car, train, or bus. When you arrive at work, you sit 8 to 10 hours in an office chair. At the end of the day, you have another seated commute back home, followed by a "sit down" dinner with family. Then perhaps you watch an hour or two of television before going to bed.

Of course, you do have a few hours of activity tucked inside this otherwise sedentary day. Yet when you look at a typical day, it is easy to see how long periods of time when you are *not in motion* can add up. The challenge is to examine each of these situations. Figure out how to slowly add a little movement, or at least spend less time sitting each day. There are literally hundreds of moments in a day when you can embed extra activity into your routine.

● ● ●

Sleep Longer to Get More Done

One less hour of sleep does not equal an extra hour of achievement or enjoyment. The exact opposite occurs. When you lose an hour of sleep, it decreases your well-being, productivity, health, and ability to think. Yet people continue to sacrifice sleep before all else.

In some workplaces, it is a badge of honor to "pull an all-nighter" to get work done. Then comes boasting about having only four hours of sleep the night before a meeting to show your colleagues just how hard you are working. I fell into this trap for many years, until I realized just how flawed this logic is from every vantage point.

One of the most influential studies of human performance, conducted by professor K. Anders Ericsson, found that elite performers need 10,000 hours of "deliberate practice" to reach levels of greatness. While this finding sparked a debate about the role of natural talent versus countless hours of practice, another element was all but missed. If you go back to Ericsson's landmark 1993 study, there was another factor that significantly influenced peak performance: sleep. On average, the best performers slept 8 hours and 36 minutes. The average American, for comparison, gets just 6 hours and 51 minutes of sleep on weeknights.

The person you want to fly your airplane, operate on your body, teach your children, or lead your organization tomorrow is the one who sleeps soundly tonight. Yet in many cases, people in these vital occupations are the ones who think they need the least sleep. And more than 30 percent of workers sleep less than six hours per night.

This sleep-related productivity loss costs about $2,000 per person a year and leads to poorer performance and lower work quality. Getting fewer than six hours of sleep a night is also the top risk factor for burnout on the job. If you want to succeed in your job, make sure your work allows you to stay in bed long enough.

Professor Ericsson's studies of elite performers — including musicians, athletes, actors, and chess players — also reveal how resting more can maximize achievement. He found that the top performers in each of these fields typically practice in focused sessions lasting no longer than 90 minutes. The best performers work in bursts. They take frequent breaks to avoid exhaustion and ensure they can recover completely. This allows them to keep going the next day.

Prevent sleeplessness from slowing you down. Working on a task too long can actually decrease your performance. To avoid this, work in bursts, take regular breaks, and make sure you get enough sleep to be productive. When you need an extra hour of energy, add an hour of sleep.

○ ○ ○

> Identify the healthiest elements of diets you have tried. Build them in to your lifestyle for good.

> Each morning, plan ahead to add activity to your daily routine.

> Sleep longer tonight to do more tomorrow.

Small Adjustments

Every Bite Is a Net Gain or Loss

Each bite you take is a small but important choice. Every sip requires another brief choice. If you make a decision that does more *good than harm*, such as opting for water over soda, it is a net gain. When you pick a side of fries instead of vegetables, it is a net loss. Even seemingly positive choices can turn into a net loss if you are not careful about everything that goes into a particular food or drink.

At one restaurant I visit regularly, the most popular entrée is the "harvest salad." Even the name sounds nutritious. Yet by the time this salad meets a fork, it is covered with small pieces of fried chicken and bacon and coated in a fat-laden ranch dressing. Good intentions, seductive label, wrong outcome.

The same thing occurs with drinks. Coffee by itself is good for you. Each sip you take is a net gain for your health. However, if you add cream and a few packets of sugar, each sip becomes a net loss. Or look at any of the packaged "green tea" drinks in a supermarket. In most cases, the added sweeteners and preservatives turn it into a much less healthy drink than real green tea.

You can modify many choices to ensure they are a net gain. One of my favorite meals is the hickory grilled salmon at a local restaurant. While it sounds healthy, I eventually realized the tasty barbecue sauce covering my filet of salmon was almost pure sugar.

After studying the nutritional content of common barbecue sauces, I realized it is essentially pancake syrup for meat. I could have told myself that the benefit of eating salmon outweighed the downside of the sugary sauce. But the only way to make this a clear net gain was to order my salmon without the barbecue sauce. A few months after making this switch, I learned to enjoy the actual taste of fresh salmon without the overpowering sauce.

There are a few good and bad ingredients in most meals. No matter how hard you try, you will eat some foods that are not ideal. But do a little accounting in your head. Ask yourself if what you are about to eat is a net gain, based on what you know about all the ingredients. If you develop a habit of asking this question, you will make better decisions in the moment.

Step Away From Your Chair

Sitting is the most underrated health threat of modern times. This subtle epidemic is eroding our health. On a global level, inactivity now kills more people than smoking.

Sitting more than six hours a day greatly increases your risk of an early death. No matter how much you exercise, eat well, avoid smoking, or add other healthy habits, excessive sitting will cause problems. Every hour you spend on your rear end — in a car, watching television, attending a meeting, or at your computer — saps your energy and ruins your health.

Sitting also makes you fat. Over the span of the last two decades, while exercise rates stayed the same, time spent sitting increased, and obesity rates doubled. One leading diabetes researcher claims that sitting for extended periods poses a health risk as "insidious" as smoking or overexposure to sunlight. He contends that physicians need to view exposure to sitting just like a skin cancer expert views exposure to direct sunlight.

"Sitting disease" also takes a toll in the moment. As soon as you sit down, electrical activity in your leg muscles shuts off. The number of calories you burn drops to one per minute. Enzyme production, which helps break down fat, drops by 90 percent.

After two hours of sitting, your good cholesterol drops by 20 percent. Perhaps this explains why people with desk jobs have twice the rate of cardiovascular disease. Or as another diabetes researcher put it, even two hours of exercise will not compensate for spending 22 hours sitting on your rear end.

Yet for many people, sitting for several hours a day is inevitable. The key is to stand, stretch, and increase activity as much as possible. Get up and move around while you're watching television. Walk to someone's office instead of calling.

Simply standing in place increases your energy more than sitting. Walking increases energy levels by about 150 percent. Taking the stairs instead of the elevator increases energy by more than 200 percent. Instead of viewing a long walk as something you don't have time for, think of it as an opportunity to get in some extra activity that will make you healthier.

◎ ◎ ◎

Sleep Makes or Breaks a Day

Missing sleep can change the trajectory of an entire week. On a recent Tuesday evening, our dog woke me up in the middle of a stormy night. She whimpered and howled for at least an hour until the rain subsided. I finally fell back to sleep at 3 a.m., only to hear my alarm blaring two hours later.

That morning, it took me longer to get out of bed. By the time I compensated with coffee, I was running behind, so I postponed my morning workout. Once I was at the office, I needed to get through countless emails, so I responded to all of them quickly with little thought. It took extra effort to focus my dry and tired eyes on the glare of the computer screen. While on conference calls, my mindset was to get through them as quickly as possible, instead of being helpful or proactive.

This cycle continued throughout the week as I struggled to catch up. Perhaps it would have been different if our dog had kept me up on a Thursday. Getting behind on a Tuesday was detrimental to my energy and interactions for several days. By the end of the week, one of my colleagues asked the dreaded "Is everything okay?" My wife and kids also felt the aftershocks of a cranky husband and dad.

You are simply a different person when you operate on insufficient sleep. And it shows. Your friends, colleagues, and loved ones can see it, even when you are too sleepless to realize your own condition. One study found that losing 90 minutes of sleep reduces daytime alertness by nearly *one-third*. If you consider all the things that demand your attention in a day, reducing alertness by one-third *is* consequential.

An extra hour of sleep could be just as essential as an additional hour of work or even another hour of physical activity. If you do not get enough sleep, it can lead to a cascade of negative events. You achieve less at work, skip regular exercise, and have poorer interactions with your loved ones.

However, if you get an additional hour of sleep, it can make the difference between a miserable day and a good one. A small adjustment, even 15 or 30 minutes, could make or break your next day. While it may seem like skipping sleep is the only way you can get other things done, doing so comes at a cost.

○ ○ ○

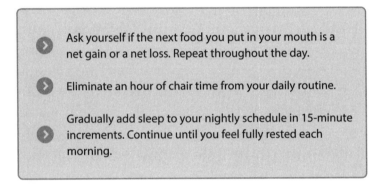

> Ask yourself if the next food you put in your mouth is a net gain or a net loss. Repeat throughout the day.

> Eliminate an hour of chair time from your daily routine.

> Gradually add sleep to your nightly schedule in 15-minute increments. Continue until you feel fully rested each morning.

What Counts More Than Calories

Reading a nutritional label and focusing on calories alone will lead you astray. While 9 percent of people read nutritional labels regularly, just *1 percent read beyond the headline of total calories*. A coffee shop in my neighborhood recently advertised lattes "under 200 calories." I fell for their clever marketing one morning and used it as an excuse to get a vanilla latte instead of regular coffee. Later on that day, I went to the coffee shop's website and realized that 150-calorie latte also has 28g of carbohydrates and a whopping 27g of sugar. This choice was not a great way to start the day, despite the relatively low calorie count.

Most people eat more carbohydrates than they need and don't get enough protein. Large-scale studies show that even modest increases in protein intake, coupled with a reduction in carbohydrates, helps us to be healthier. If you look at the nutritional label on most packaged foods, you will notice the total grams (g) of carbohydrates outnumber the grams of protein in a serving. In most cases, the carbs greatly outweigh the protein, by 10 to 1 or higher.

Instead of focusing on total calories, another simple way to screen all the options you see in a day is to look at the ratio of carbs to protein. Set a goal of eating foods that have a *ratio of one gram of carbs for every one gram of protein*. I started doing this several years ago, and it is a great shortcut when scanning items in a grocery store or restaurant. Almost every nutritional label I found lists both the total carbohydrates and total protein. For example, the mixed nuts I snack on regularly, the avocado salad I order for lunch, and my favorite Indian meal (palak paneer) all sit right at or near a 1 to 1 ratio.

At a minimum, avoid foods with a ratio higher than 5 to 1 carbs to protein. Most snack chips and cereals have a 10 to 1 ratio. Maintaining a better balance of carbohydrates to protein will give you additional energy while improving your health in the long run. Using this 1 to 1 ratio may not be the perfect metric for evaluating food, but it is a decent shortcut to ensuring that you are not overloading on carbs.

Use Product Placement at Home

Marketers have known for decades that you buy what you see first. You are far more likely to purchase items placed at eye level in the grocery store, for example, than items on the bottom shelf. There is an entire body of research about the way "product placement" in stores influences your buying behavior.

This gives you a chance to use product placement to your advantage. Healthy items like produce are often the least visible foods at home. You won't think to eat what you don't see. This may be part of the reason why 85 percent of Americans do not eat enough fruits and vegetables.

If produce is hidden in a drawer at the bottom of your refrigerator, these good foods are out of sight and mind. The same holds true for your pantry. I used to have a shelf lined with salty crackers and chips at eye level. When these were the first things I noticed, they were my primary snack foods. That same shelf is now filled with healthy snacks, which makes good decisions easy.

Foods that sit out on tables and countertops are even more critical. When you see food every time you walk by, it gives you permission to graze. So to improve your choices, leave good foods like apples and pistachios sitting out instead of crackers and candy.

Go through the places in your house where you store food. Organize items so the *best choices* are the *first things you see* and the easiest to reach. Then hide poor choices in inconvenient places where you might not see them for a while. Better yet, simply clean house and discard foods with little nutritional value you know you'll be tempted to eat.

Move fruits, vegetables, and other healthy options closer to eye level in your refrigerator or put them out on a counter. Simply seeing fresh produce regularly will plant a seed in your mind for your next snack. This also gives you a head start at resisting temptation in the moment.

● ● ●

Work Faster While You Walk

Working on this book was an experiment in itself. While I had read a fair amount of research about the downside of sitting, I read most of it ... sitting down. To make things even more difficult, because I have written several books, I know it requires even longer periods sitting at my desk than normal. It's no coincidence my back pain is always at its worst when I am writing and editing. What's more, a recent study found a strong association between long-term sedentary work and rates of cancer.

Given the topic of this book, it was time for a new approach. I decided to build a workstation on my treadmill and set a goal of writing this entire book while walking. So I mounted my computer monitor above my treadmill and built a homemade keyboard tray across the arm rests.

Because it was a low-cost solution, I figured it was worth trying even if it did not work out.

Initially, I didn't know if it would be possible to type, look at my screen, and use a touchpad while in motion. A few days into the experiment, I determined that as long as I maintain a pace of 1.5 miles per hour, it worked. At this pace, I can read, type, and talk on the phone at least as easily as if I were seated. When I use voice dictation software for extended periods of writing, I am able to write far more words per day than I can when I'm seated.

After using this homemade walking desk for several months, I am now walking *an additional 5-10 miles per day* as a result. At the end of each "walk day," as I have started to call it, my back no longer aches. I also have dramatically more energy compared with days when I am sitting in meetings, cars, or airplanes.

By the time this book was nearing publication, a wide range of commercial options had emerged for working while walking, standing, or a mix of standing and sitting. One of the most common treadmill brands now produces a model with an integrated desk for a keyboard and monitor. It gets even better reviews from users than the model without a built-in desk. A recumbent bicycle with an integrated laptop desk is even more popular. This "pedal desk" will set you back about $250, which is reasonable in the context of how much it could contribute to your health.

If it is remotely practical, try something like this to increase activity, even if it's only when you are at home. I have a friend who forces himself to watch sporting events while on his elliptical machine, so he is getting a little activity alongside his favorite athletes. Another option is a standing desk or a convertible desk that moves up and down for standing *and* seated work.

If you stand still while you work, it is a good idea to alternate between standing and sitting. Standing still for extended periods can cause unnecessary strain if you don't move around or alternate with sitting. You can also find adapters that secure to a stationary desk and allow you to raise and lower your monitor and keyboard to a standing or seated level.

All of these options are gaining popularity in workplaces as companies discover the cost savings from fewer sick days associated with excessive sitting. Several organizations I have worked with provide shared walking workstations where employees can go to catch up on email. I spoke with a friend the other day who used one of these shared workstations to complete all of his annual online compliance training.

If your employer will not provide walking or standing desks (it never hurts to ask), put your laptop or monitor on a shelf where you can stand and work occasionally. Or get a music stand, wall mount, or something that makes it easy to read and work while standing. At a minimum, try

reading on a stationary bike, or take a walk while listening
to an audio book or conference call.

○ ○ ○

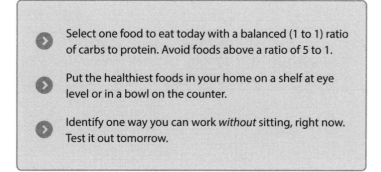

Select one food to eat today with a balanced (1 to 1) ratio
of carbs to protein. Avoid foods above a ratio of 5 to 1.

Put the healthiest foods in your home on a shelf at eye
level or in a bowl on the counter.

Identify one way you can work *without* sitting, right now.
Test it out tomorrow.

Sugar Is the Next Nicotine

Sugar is a toxin. It fuels diabetes, obesity, heart disease, and cancer. At the current dose we consume, more than 150 pounds per person *every year*, sugar and its derivatives kill more people than cocaine, heroin, or any other controlled substance.

One report aptly described sugar as "candy for cancer cells." It accelerates aging and inflammation in the body and subsequently fuels tumor growth. It is now clear that if you lower your sugar intake, you reduce the odds of cancer.

As additional research emerges, even higher "normal" glucose levels (82 to 110 mg/dL) have an adverse impact on your health over time. Blood sugar levels at the higher end of the normal range have been linked to significant shrinkage of the brain. The more sugar you consume, the greater the levels of inflammation in your body. This leads you to age faster, inside and out. There is simply no good reason to consume any *added* sugars beyond what you get from whole fruits and vegetables.

People once thought of smoking a cigarette as a pleasant break. It relieved stress, satisfied a craving, and provided a quick high. Sound familiar? Then we learned smoking creates cumulative damage in our bodies, causes cancer, makes us look older, and decreases our energy. People finally started to kick the habit, as hard as it may be.

Much like cigarettes, sugars are addictive. Each time you eat sweets, it causes your brain to light up, produce dopamine, and want more sugar. In the words of one leading neuroscientist, sweets "fire the reward regions in our brain" much like other drugs. Your brain also builds a tolerance to sugar over time, one that mirrors the way people habituate to alcohol or tobacco. As a result, once you consume sugar, your body needs larger quantities over time to mimic the pleasurable sensation.

This is why drug companies are now scrambling to find compounds that reduce the body's normal uptake of sugar. Their goal is to produce pills you can take every day to counteract your cravings for sugar, thus reducing the odds of heart disease, diabetes, and cancer. Yet like a nicotine gum or patch, this is a temporary solution. Over time, you need to wean yourself off added sugars.

Eliminating *all* sugar from your diet tomorrow is about as realistic as telling a lifetime smoker to go cold turkey. It might be even harder because sugars are embedded in so many foods, products, events, and celebrations. Sugar also has an unfair advantage; it manipulates our brains so we consume larger amounts over time.

Yet you have a responsibility to defend yourself. Start by cutting back on *added* sugar. Added sugar is not just the packets you pour into your tea or coffee. In most cases, sugar is already in the prepared and packaged foods you consume.

Study nutritional labels and look for the total grams (g) of sugar. The closer to zero the better. Any packaged product with more than 10g of sugar is more than you need in a single serving. While the American Heart Association recommends limiting added sugar intake to 25g (6 teaspoons a day) for women and 38g (9 teaspoons a day) for men, a better goal is to keep your daily total in the single digits. Remember, there is absolutely no nutritional need for foods with added sugars.

○ ○ ○

Substitutes Are a Nicotine Patch

If you have a sweet tooth, it's not your fault. Generations ago, a preference for sweet tastes was coded into your genes for the sake of survival. Foods that *naturally* contain fructose are not poisonous. This provided your distant ancestors with a way to avoid eating things in the wild that threatened their survival. Over time, the preference for sweet taste was built into your genes. As a result, you are born to trust any sweet taste as safe.

While sweet-tasting foods will not kill you immediately, this preference no longer serves your evolutionary instinct to survive. You can forget the debate about which sugar derivative or substitute is "less bad for you." Anything that makes your food or drink taste sweet leads you to crave less healthy foods later. So even if you believe that the latest organic, safe-for-diabetics sweetener is okay for your health, it will still work against you in the long run. Once a sweet taste hits your tongue, it sets a cycle in motion, and you consume even more sugar by the hour.

I used to add a sugar substitute and creamer to my coffee every morning. After a few cups, I would crave sweet tastes later in the day as well. On most days, I would have a couple of diet sodas and a sugary snack in the afternoon. Then a few years ago, I decided to eliminate the artificial sweetener from my coffee. I also replaced the sweetened creamer with unsweetened coconut milk, which eliminated any sweet taste from my morning routine. This made it remarkably easy to avoid diet soda and sugary snacks later.

Look at your own daily routine. Consider what you could do to curb sugar cravings early in the day. The ingredients to watch out for on labels include: agave nectar, aspartame, corn syrup, dextrose, fructose, fruit juice concentrates, high fructose corn syrup, honey, maltitol, saccharine, sorbitol, stevia, sucrose, sucralose, and sugar. While some of these options are probably better than others, the more you avoid any added sweetener, the fewer subsequent cravings you will have for sugary foods.

If you consume fewer sugars and substitutes, your body will see a rapid benefit. New research shows how reducing the amount of fructose you consume can lead to major changes in as little as two weeks. As you reduce this biological desire for sweet tastes over time, you will need significantly less willpower to pass on the cake.

● ● ●

Take Two Every Twenty

The act of sitting literally makes your backside bigger. When researchers studied MRI images of muscle tissue, they found that sitting around for long periods of time could put pressure on cells and cause the body to produce 50 percent more fat than it usually would. This research suggests that when force is placed on a specific area in the body for an extended time, it causes fat tissue to expand. So even if you exercise regularly, sitting for many hours encourages fat cells to congregate near your rear.

When you have no choice but to sit for several hours a day, at least break it up. If you sit for hours on end, your blood sugar and insulin levels will spike to dangerous levels. However, taking regular breaks can counterbalance these spikes. In experimental settings, even two minutes of leisurely walking every 20 minutes was enough to stabilize blood sugar levels.

If getting up and moving around regularly is not natural for you, trick yourself into being active. Do something to remind yourself to get up at least two or three times per hour. One way to force movement is to increase your consumption of liquid. This makes you get up more often for refills and restroom breaks.

A colleague of mine who tends to get focused and lose track of time when he works at his computer uses a timer on his smartphone. He sets the timer to play a subtle audible alert every 20 minutes. This reminds him to take a quick break, walk around the office, stand up, or stretch.

Don't worry about breaks every 20 minutes ruining your focus on a task. Contrary to what I might have guessed, taking regular breaks from mental tasks actually improves your creativity and productivity. Skipping breaks, on the other hand, leads to stress and fatigue. As one management professor described, mental concentration is akin to a muscle that gets fatigued with prolonged use. It needs a period of rest before it can recover. Getting up for the sake of your body may yield as much benefit for your mind.

Also examine your surroundings and think about how you can prevent sedentary time. We've built our lives around convenience, so anything we need is within arms' reach. This translates into sitting for longer periods without having to get up, move, and interact with other people. Instead, organize your home and office to encourage movement over convenience.

○ ○ ○

> Identify the sugar content in your favorite meal or snack. If it's more than 10g, find a replacement.

> Pick one food or drink you sweeten regularly — artificially or with sugar — and consume it without the added sweetener for a week.

> When you have to sit for long periods of time, stand up, walk, or stretch every 20 minutes.

Judge Food by the Color of Its Skin

The benefit of a diet rich in fruits and vegetables is so well-documented it hardly bears repeating. Eating the right natural foods wards off disease, enables you to live longer, makes you look better, and gives you additional energy. Yet most people fail to eat enough fruits and vegetables but consume large quantities of unnecessary foods.

This problem influences more than just your physical health. A study of 80,000+ people suggests that total intake of fruits and vegetables is a robust predictor of overall happiness. Every additional daily serving of fruits or vegetables, all the way up to seven servings, continues to improve well-being.

However, we do not have a quick way to determine what foods are the healthiest. We receive conflicting advice from different sources. Then we face countless choices every time we go to a grocery store or place an order at a restaurant.

An efficient mental shortcut is to judge a fruit or vegetable by the color of its skin. Generally speaking, produce with dark and vibrant colors is your best bet. Green means go. Broccoli, spinach, kale, bok choy, celery, cucumbers, peppers, zucchini, and other dark leafy greens are net positives for your health. Also look to red or blue fruits and vegetables as good nutritional sources. Apples, peppers, raspberries, strawberries, tomatoes, and almost any fruit or vegetable with vibrant skin tone makes for a better choice.

The next time you are in a grocery store, start by shopping in sections with dark-colored fruits and vegetables. Spend as much time as possible in the produce section before loading up on other foods. When you get home, prepare your plate with dark and diverse colors. When you dine out, ask for greens instead of grains. Order what you would normally put on a sandwich on top of spinach or romaine.

● ● ●

A Vaccine for the Common Cold

Getting a flu shot every year takes some forward thinking. The flu is usually a risk in the distance versus an immediate threat. The shot requires a little pain today in hopes of preventing a lot more misery in the future. This challenge is part of the reason why millions of people don't get vaccinated each year. What if someone told you there was finally a vaccine for the common cold? One that requires no painful injection or doctor visit, yet is even more effective at preventing a cold than a flu shot is against influenza.

One experiment suggests a good night's sleep may be the answer. Participants in this study reported their sleep quality for 14 consecutive nights. Then they were quarantined and given nasal drops containing a rhinovirus (common cold). Researchers monitored participants for the next five days to see if they developed a cold. This experiment revealed that the participants who typically had less than seven hours of sleep before being exposed to the rhinovirus were nearly *three times as likely to develop a cold*.

Even though you cannot see it, a sound night's sleep alters what is going on inside your body. Sleep deprivation raises blood pressure, increases inflammation, and boosts the risk of heart disease and stroke. These outcomes suggest sleep is an even higher priority when you are likely to catch a cold or the flu.

During cold and flu season, for example, your immune system may need enough sleep to ward off the latest strain going around your office. When your sleep routine is at risk, due to travel or any other reason, plan your schedule to get the right amount of sleep. This will keep your natural defenses high when you are at an increased risk of getting sick.

○ ○ ○

Quality Beats Quantity in Bed

It is easy to spend eight hours in bed and still feel lousy in the morning. There are many nights when I spend more than eight hours in bed but get far fewer hours of quality sleep. To study this in more depth, I tested a sophisticated sleep-tracking device to get a better gauge of my sleep quality.

The device I used consisted of a headband with a large sensor that sat in the middle of my forehead at night. This sensor communicated with a special alarm clock on my nightstand. Every morning when I got out of bed, my alarm clock would display a total sleep quality number. It also gave me detailed information about how long I was in bed but still awake as well as my time in light sleep, deep sleep, and REM sleep.

I was only able to test this device for a few weeks because my wife threatened to take a picture of me wearing the ridiculous-looking headband and share it with friends. However, I learned all I needed to know. In short, my detailed sleep quality scores matched my own subjective rating of my sleep almost perfectly. When I was up most of the night stressed out about something, my sleep quality was markedly lower. On mornings when I felt well-rested, my sleep quality score was near-perfect.

It was also clear from my experience that total time in bed is not the right number to watch. You can spend nine hours in bed yet get just five hours of good sleep. The problem is, time spent rolling around awake in bed doesn't count. Nor is it healthy if you are regularly getting up in the middle of the night and struggling to fall back to sleep.

As part of the experiment in the previous section in which people were quarantined and injected with a rhinovirus, participants were also graded on the *quality* or efficiency of their sleep. To determine the "sleep efficiency" scores for each participant, researchers asked what time they went to sleep, what time they got up, how much time they spent in bed before falling asleep, how many times they awoke, and how long they were up throughout the night. The sleep efficiency score was then calculated based on the percentage of time participants slept out of the total time they were in bed.

The researchers discovered that sleep efficiency is more influential than the total duration of sleep, at least when it comes to warding off the common cold. Participants who had lower sleep efficiency scores over the 14-day period before exposure to the rhinovirus were *5.5 times as likely to develop a cold*. Quality of sleep beat quantity by a wide margin.

Set yourself up for quality sleep first. Consider your diet, activity, and environment. Then focus on extending how long you sleep.

○ ○ ○

> Every time you go to the store, start by loading up on fruits and vegetables with vibrant colors.

> When disruptions threaten your regular schedule, plan ahead to ensure you get a good night's sleep.

> As you make adjustments for better sleep, measure your progress. Note the time you get into bed and the time you wake up. Then rate your sleep quality on a 1-10 scale.

What Counts

Wear a New Pair of Genes

Bad genes are no excuse for an unhealthy lifestyle. As I mentioned at the beginning of this book, I have a rare condition that is the equivalent of losing the genetic lottery. Yet the worst thing I could do is blame my genes and use them as an excuse to make poor choices. If I were to go through life blaming "bad genes" and playing the role of a victim, it would make things far worse.

As scientists are now uncovering, your lifestyle choices can create rapid and dramatic changes at the genetic level. Even with a family history of obesity or heart disease, you will benefit from a better diet, more activity, and quality sleep. Lifestyle choices can be even more influential than your genetic background. Simply being active is associated with a 40 percent reduction in the genetic predisposition for obesity, according to a study of more than 20,000 adults. While your genes can make it easier to become obese, they do not prevent you from being healthy.

Another experiment showed how participants who underwent just three months of major lifestyle adjustments, from diet to exercise, created changes in the activity of about 500 genes. There was more activity in disease-preventing genes and less activity in disease-promoting genes. One of the strongest genetic mutations for heart disease can even be altered. High fruit and vegetable intake almost negates the effect of this mutation that predisposes people to cardiovascular disease.

While you will not be able to change your genes altogether, you clearly can alter the expression of your genes and the subsequent impact they have on your health over time. You obviously can't change your family history. However, you *can change your family future* by making better choices today.

⊙ ⊙ ⊙

Measuring Makes You Move More

In 2008, I ordered a small gadget called a Fitbit to measure my daily steps and activity. The device is about the size of a tube of lip balm. All I have to do is clip it to my waist or put it in my pocket. Whenever I walk past a wireless sensor, the device uploads my data to a website. It also shows my total steps on a small digital display so I can check my progress throughout the day. At the time, this was a revolutionary way to track steps, miles walked, and what percentage of my day was active.

When I started tracking my progress, I was walking only two miles a day. After tracking this metric for more than four years, I now walk at least five miles, even on a slow day. If I had not started measuring my daily steps and miles, there is no way I would be as active today.

One little secret of medicine and social sciences is how *measurement itself creates improvement*. When researchers study the effect of a given intervention, simply asking people to track a specific outcome makes it more likely to improve. While this is a limitation for scientific experiments, you can use this to your advantage.

If you want to increase your activity, measure how much you move. When people are assigned to wear a pedometer as part of randomized controlled trials, they walk at least one *extra mile* per day on average. Overall activity levels go up by 27 percent. Body Mass Index (BMI) decreases, and blood pressure goes down.

In addition to basic pedometers, which cost as little as $5, more sophisticated tools are available today. There are now hundreds of devices that can measure your activity all day long. They come in the form of wristbands, necklaces, GPS watches, and other clip-on or in-pocket devices.

Some of these tools even monitor the duration and quality of your sleep. Others track your heart rate and alert you if you are inactive for a prolonged period. You can also achieve much of this using the accelerometer or GPS in a smartphone. All you need to do is download an app.

If you have the slightest interest in gadgets, this is a golden era for health-based information. These devices are easy to use and relatively inexpensive. An entire industry is emerging around this "quantified self" movement. Even if you're not into technology, you can always map your walk, run, or commute to calculate the total distance. When you start to measure, the improvement will come.

Whether you prefer high tech, low tech, or no tech, find some way to track or log your activity. This will prompt you to set specific goals — yet another key to adding movement. What could be even more beneficial is comparing your activity levels to your peers' activity levels. At a minimum, tracking your activity keeps it top of mind.

○ ○ ○

Target 10,000

Once you find a way to measure your movement, set a goal for your daily activity. The most common standard is the raw number of steps you take in a day. Almost any pedometer or device tracks and displays your total steps.

When I first started counting, my typical day was just 5,000 steps. Until I received this daily feedback, I had no idea how sedentary my lifestyle had become. After tracking continuously for a year, I was hitting 8,000 steps per day on average, and I now routinely walk more than 10,000 steps a day. Every night, the last thing I look at before bed is my step count for the day. This number is a decent proxy for whether my body had a good day or a rough one.

Based on the latest research, 10,000 steps per day is a good target for overall activity. This equates to roughly five miles, which is nowhere near as daunting as it sounds once you start adding up all of your daily movement. On the other end of the continuum, people who walk fewer than 5,500 steps are considered sedentary.

When researchers compared average number of steps per day across different nations, they discovered that the average American falls below this sedentary line at just 5,117 steps per day. In comparison, the average Australian takes 9,695 steps per day, nearly two times the average American's steps per day. This helps explain why Australia's obesity rate is just 16 percent, while the United States' is 34 percent.

The good news is, going from the lower end of this continuum to the recommended 10,000 steps leads to significant health benefits — from weight loss to warding off diabetes. Start doing smaller things each day to increase your total. If you live in a city, walk to the *second* closest coffee shop. Instead of trolling for the parking spot right by an entrance, find one at the back of the lot.

Try to get a few hundred steps around your home or office every hour. Take a brisk walk during your lunch break for 30 minutes, which could add about 3,000 steps. Play an active sport for an hour to add 8,000-10,000 steps. Then if you have a day when you just can't get to 10,000, aim for a weekly total of at least 70,000 to balance things out.

○ ○ ○

> Build your meals around fruits and vegetables today to change the expression of your genes tomorrow.

> Select one way to measure your daily movement. Use a pedometer, watch, GPS, smartphone, or manual log to start tracking your activity today.

> Aim for 10,000 steps every day or 70,000 steps per week.

Refined Fuel

Be Less Refined

We are addicted to refined carbohydrates. They are a staple of most meals. People put carbs in a bowl for breakfast, slap two pieces of bread around protein for lunch, and allow carbs to overwhelm their dinner plate. Much like sugars, the more refined carbs — such as white bread or white rice — you consume, the more you crave them throughout the day.

All carbohydrates convert to sugar in your bloodstream. The more refined they are, the faster this conversion occurs. If you eat a roll before dinner, its carbohydrates turn into blood sugar soon after entering your bloodstream.

One publication went as far as to describe carbs as "more addictive than cocaine" and concluded, "At the center of the obesity universe lies carbohydrates, not fat."

As a team of Harvard researchers wrote in the *Journal of the American Medical Association*, carbs are a "nutrient for which humans have no absolute requirement." Another study suggests that eating fewer carbs even curbs cancer growth rates by as much as 50 percent.

Yet quitting carbs altogether would be an uphill climb. Most animals, humans included, evolved to prefer the taste of carbohydrates over protein. Carbs also stimulate pleasurable dopamine centers in the brain. And they are cheap and convenient. Everywhere you turn, pasta, bread, chips, or a bowl of rice is staring you in the face. I guess this explains why it is still so hard for me to choose a salad over a sandwich.

Do everything you can to replace *refined* carbohydrates with vegetables when you prepare or order a meal. You get enough carbohydrates from fruits, vegetables, and protein. Try to reduce your consumption of pasta, bread, rice, and chips in particular. Most restaurants will let you substitute a vegetable for a side of rice, pasta, or fries. Keep most of the refined carbs from making it to your plate in the first place. That way you won't need a superhuman amount of willpower to resist what is sitting in front of you during a meal.

Watch out for all the hidden sugars and carbs in packaged snacks and snack bars as well. Last year, I got hooked on an "all-natural" almond crunch snack. Then I realized *the only way you get something to stick together and crunch is to bind it with a sugary substance*. Even the organic granola bars we had at home contained 30g of sugar, 23g of carbs, and a mere 3g of protein. As I looked closer at the items in my local grocery store aisle, almost every protein bar and so-called health snack I found was loaded with sugar or refined carbs.

Instead of chips, crackers, or bars, find natural snacks like nuts, carrots, apples, celery, kale chips, or seeds. Then avoid the processed and refined carbs at all costs. Remember, this is one case where "refined" does not mean "better" or "improved."

○ ○ ○

Family Style Is Making Us Fat

When food is served "family style" from large plates, bowls, or platters placed in arms' reach, people simply eat more. One study found that women eat about 10 percent more. Men move even faster through their first helping and *eat an additional 29 percent* if the dish is on the table instead of on the counter.

Family style starts out with good intentions. When you prepare a meal for a group of people, you fix more food to make sure there is enough for everyone.

But the large serving plates moving around the table create peer pressure. Everyone feels obligated to take a sample of each item to avoid offending the chef. Then, everyone sits around with more food within reach, making it far too easy to grab seconds or even thirds.

To avoid eating more food than you need, leave the serving plates in the kitchen, on a counter, or anywhere else that requires people to stand up and leave the table for another helping. This will allow your family and friends to be selective and take only what they really want. It should also keep them from eating too much and becoming uncomfortably full.

Once you move the serving plates off the table, you might notice that people are less likely to get up and grab seconds or thirds. Some people will remain seated just to avoid the perception of overeating. Others will stay seated simply because getting up requires effort. Either way, sit back and watch how you have channeled social pressure in a positive direction.

Also, when you cook for yourself or your immediate family and you make extra food to save for leftovers, put those portions away before you eat. If you leave the excess food sitting out, someone is bound to eat more than they had originally planned.

This small and easy change makes a real difference. After testing this myself over the last year, I now put less on my plate to start with and rarely go back to the kitchen for a second serving. All it takes is a little planning before you sit down to eat. The rest is almost automatic.

● ● ●

Burn Calories *After* Your Workout

While a few hours of activity a day sounds like a daunting challenge, it is not when you reverse the equation. If someone told you to avoid 23 hours of inactivity per day, I assume you would agree with this advice wholeheartedly. Yet without some deliberate effort, it is easy to spend 23 hours a day sitting, sleeping, and moving slowly.

A few years ago, I began tracking the percentage of time I was active in a given day. I always considered myself to be someone who leads an active lifestyle. But it turned out nearly 20 hours of my day was occupied by sleeping, sitting, and being lightly active. Then about three hours was just fairly active, or the equivalent of walking.

That left well under an hour of very active time, when I was getting real cardiovascular activity. As I studied these patterns, I realized how important it was to first move as much time as possible away from the completely sedentary category. Then I increased my amount of very active time by walking briskly, running, and biking.

Study your distribution of activity for one of your typical days. Start with the easy math and add up how much time you spend sitting each day. Do everything possible to reduce that number. Then focus on doing anything that gets your heart beating a little faster than normal.

Any workout will burn calories. However, as your level of intensity increases, you continue burning calories for many hours after your workout ends. New research suggests that vigorous activity could increase the total benefit of a workout by nearly 50 percent over the duration of an entire day. When participants in an experiment rode a stationary bicycle at high intensity for 45 minutes, the exercise itself burned about 420 calories. Yet what is most interesting is that over the next 14 hours, the participants burned 190 additional calories on average.

When you exercise, push yourself to the point where it would be hard to have a conversation. Or use a heart rate monitor to ensure you are in the right target zone. If you can get to this point for much of the workout, your body will continue to benefit for hours after you exercise.

○ ○ ○

> Replace chips, crackers, and snack bars with nuts, seeds, apples, celery, and carrots.

> Always leave the serving dishes in the kitchen; don't bring them to the table.

> Get a full hour of vigorous activity to burn calories all day long.

Empty Stomach, Bad Choices

The hungrier you are, the harder it is to resist unhealthy foods. When your stomach is empty, your blood sugar levels drop. This increases your desire for foods like burgers, pizza, brownies, and ice cream. When researchers used functional MRI brain scans to study why this happens, they discovered that the body focuses on feeding itself high-calorie foods to get blood sugar levels back to normal.

An empty stomach also makes you more likely to start your meal with the wrong foods, even when you have a variety of choices. One experiment found that students who were asked to fast from dinner until lunch the next day were more than *two times* as likely to start their meal with a roll or french fries, compared with a control group that ate normally. In contrast, most of the people in the control group started by eating a vegetable.

Perhaps you have experienced this before. You haven't eaten in a while, and you are starting to get hungry. As time passes, almost any food is appealing, healthy or not. If you give in to temptation, you eat more than normal. I know my willpower falls apart if I have not had anything to eat for several hours. This leads me to eat about anything I can find. I also consume more and at a faster pace when my stomach is running on empty.

Several years ago, I realized this was taking a toll on my health. If I got hungry on a long drive, I stopped at the nearest fast-food restaurant. When rushing through an airport, I would grab a sandwich or energy bar for my flight. Anytime I was hungry *and* in a hurry, it resulted in a bad choice.

To keep myself from going into starvation mode, I decided to keep a standby pack of mixed nuts in my work bag. This homemade snack pack now goes everywhere with me, just in case I am stuck with no healthy options nearby. Not only does this help satisfy cravings, it also serves as a backup when I attend meetings or events with limited food choices.

When you are away from home, take small bags of nuts, fruits, or vegetables with you in case you get hungry. Keep these healthy snacks nearby to satisfy a mid-afternoon craving. When you plan for healthier choices in advance, poor last-minute decisions are easy to avoid.

○ ○ ○

The 20-Minute Meal Rule

Given my lack of patience, I know how easy it is to devour a meal in five minutes, particularly when I'm in a rush. For most of my life, I have viewed eating as one more thing I need to complete as quickly as possible. This made fast food and microwavable meals two of my best friends when I was growing up.

When I first got married and went to dinner with my in-laws, I remember how frustrating it was when they took a full hour to eat their meal. As much as I enjoyed the company and conversation between bites, I found myself sitting with a clean plate for the last 45 minutes of each meal, looking at everyone else around the table as their forks moved between the plate and their mouth in what felt like slow motion. As it turns out, my in-laws had it right.

The more I studied this topic, the more I learned that nothing good comes from racing through meals. When you eat too fast, your digestive system does not have enough time to send a "you're getting full" message to your brain. So you tend to keep eating — and end up eating too much. When you overeat, you get less enjoyment from consuming the excess quantities compared with the initial flavorful bites. So when you rush through a meal, you eat more than you need, and you enjoy the food less.

Eating fast not only leads to overconsumption, but it also nearly doubles your risk of obesity and increases your odds of Type 2 diabetes by two and a half times. In contrast, if you eat slowly and take the time to savor each bite, you will consume significantly less and avoid these ill effects.

Rapid eating can also cause discomfort after a meal. When you eat too fast, you introduce extra air into your digestive tract. This overloads your stomach, causing it to produce more acid. The result is heartburn, or what is technically known as gastroesophageal reflux disease (GERD). One study found that eating a meal in 5 rather than 30 minutes made people 50 percent more likely to have heartburn.

In contrast, an extended meal with friends is one of the best investments of your time for a variety of reasons. Take time to enjoy each bite of food along with the conversation. Spend more time with loved ones, eat slower, and savor the taste of your food.

If you chew your food properly, *a meal should take at least 20 minutes*, according to one expert. Slowing down can also give your brain and stomach time to realize you are getting full. I find the 20-minute rule to be a good general guideline, especially when I eat alone. Although I am still tempted to eat much faster, aiming for 20 minutes at least slows me down.

Even when takeout food is the only option, there are things you can do to slow your consumption. Something as simple as forcing yourself to put your food, arm, fork, or spoon down between bites can help you avoid rapidly shoveling food into your mouth. Savor the first few bites of each meal. Learn to enjoy the *process* of eating foods that are good for you.

○ ○ ○

Move Early for a 12-Hour Mood Boost

Trust me, I have made every excuse in the book for not working out in the morning: early meeting, long commute, or getting kids to school. Yet the reality is, you are the only one who misses out if you don't exercise first thing in the morning.

When a team of researchers assigned a group of college students to exercise, then tracked their mood the next day, they made a surprising discovery. After just 20 minutes of a moderate-intensity workout, the students were in a much better mood compared with a control group of students who did not exercise. The researchers expected this result based on previous findings. What surprised them was the *durability* of this increase in mood. Students in the group who exercised continued to feel better throughout the day. They were in a better mood 2, 4, 8, and even 12 hours later.

A mere 20 minutes of moderate activity could significantly improve your mood for the next 12 hours. So, while working out in the evening is better than no activity at all, you essentially sleep through and miss most of the boost in your mood. Exercising *before* you eat breakfast, instead of after, could also burn additional fat and improve glucose tolerance. Working out early also alleviates any guilt of putting it off and provides extra energy for the remainder of the day.

After reading some of this research, I started forcing myself to exercise first thing in the morning, even when it was inconvenient. I soon realized my morning workout was essential on days when I had critical work, meetings, or presentations. On a recent two-day trip to give a speech in San Francisco, I made sure my flights were timed so I could stay on schedule and get a good night of sleep. My presentation started at 8 a.m., so I went to bed and woke up early to have time for a run and a healthy breakfast before getting ready. This kept my internal body clock on schedule and ensured I had plenty of energy for my speech.

Instead of treating morning exercise as something that will drain your energy, as it often does the first few days until you establish a routine, remember that it will eventually give you additional energy. In addition to looking and feeling better, research suggests you will have extra brainpower and creative thought following periods of vigorous activity. Working out in the morning will also keep the 12-hour mood boost from going to waste.

○ ○ ○

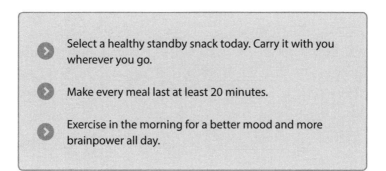

Select a healthy standby snack today. Carry it with you wherever you go.

Make every meal last at least 20 minutes.

Exercise in the morning for a better mood and more brainpower all day.

The First Order Anchors the Table

The more people you dine with, the more food you are likely to eat. When dining with one person, people eat 35 percent more than when they are alone. Sharing a meal with more than four people increases consumption by 75 percent. When people eat in groups of seven or more, they eat 96 percent more than when they dine alone. When you dine with friends, social expectations shape your decisions more than you realize.

"Anchoring" is a term behavioral scientists use to describe how people rely too heavily on the first piece of information they hear. If someone offers you a product for $100, you will think it is a deal to purchase that product for $75. With almost any purchase, small or large, the sticker price serves as an anchor for all discounts and negotiations.

The same phenomenon occurs when you dine out with friends. The first person to announce what he or she is ordering sets an anchor for the entire group. If the first person ordering chooses a healthy option, it puts a little pressure on everyone else at the table to do the same.

But if the first person to order picks the fried chicken, it makes everyone else want to give in to temptation and splurge. Research has shown how people use this "it's not as bad as what she ordered" mentality to justify poor choices. Then consider another pivotal moment — when your waiter asks if anyone wants to see the dessert menu. In most cases, we look at each other for visual cues, and then someone makes the decision about whether to accept the menu. If the first person to respond agrees to see the dessert menu, the server will bring menus for everyone at the table. Even if you had not originally planned to order dessert, you may give in.

The next time you are dining out with a group, see if you can detect how your choices influence others. If you are planning to order a healthier item, share that choice with friends while you are looking at the menu. Or be the first one to order and anchor others' decisions toward better choices.

◎ ◎ ◎

Realign Your Spine

When the wheels of a car are not aligned properly, it pulls toward one side instead of moving straight ahead. Over time, this poor alignment creates uneven wear on the car's tires. A similar problem occurs when your body's motions are not aligned and balanced. Using one side of your body far more than the other, for example, can create uneven wear and serious back problems over time.

If you don't have back pain today, you probably will at some point. The more sedentary we become and as electronic devices invade our lives, the likelihood of our spines worsening over time increases. And for those of us with chronic back issues, the smallest of incidents, such as tying a shoelace, can set off a chain of painful events.

As one spinal surgeon put it, be careful to avoid bending, lifting, and twisting in particular. During these three motions, your spine is the most vulnerable to injury. When you need to bend down and pick something up, use your knees instead of your back. Straighten up and protect your back at all times, even when you sneeze. Try not to overextend when you reach.

If you need to carry a purse or bag for more than a block, switch the side you carry it on frequently, or use a backpack to distribute the load evenly. I have noticed it helps when I alternate sides when I carry my kids. Even when I walk home from the grocery store, I now carry two lighter bags instead of one heavy bag in my dominant hand.

When you use a computer, check the basic alignment of your keyboard, screen, and chair. Then mix it up to minimize repetitive motion. If you have used your right hand to operate your mouse for years, try using your left hand.

I went as far as to put trackpads on the left and right side of my computer to force myself to use both arms interchangeably. Doing this for a few years eliminated my chronic wrist and shoulder pain. Another option is to alternate between a trackpad, trackball, touchscreen, or other input device instead of solely relying on a mouse using your dominant hand.

Apply the same principle to your phone. Switch the hand you use or the ear you speak into regularly. Do whatever you can to create variance and keep both sides of your body in balance.

○ ○ ○

Fight the Light at Night

Keep artificial light before bedtime from ruining your sleep. Exposure to light in the hours before you go to sleep suppresses melatonin levels. Lower melatonin levels make it hard to fall asleep, decrease sleep quality, and could even increase the risk of high blood pressure and diabetes.

Melatonin plays a critical role in regulating our sleeping and waking cycles. To study fluctuations in melatonin levels, one team of researchers followed 116 healthy volunteers for five consecutive days. The researchers inserted an intravenous catheter into each person's forearm. This allowed them to measure melatonin levels continuously. They discovered that exposure to bright light before bedtime decreased the beneficial effect of melatonin by 90 minutes compared with dim light exposure.

One implication from this emerging research is to consider your use of indoor lighting. Open the blinds and keep lighting bright *during the day*. Use "cool white" light bulbs near 6500K in color temperature, which are designed to mimic natural daylight, in areas where you work. These bulbs emit additional light from the blue part of the spectrum versus the yellowish light from traditional incandescent bulbs. This blue-toned electrical light and natural sunlight slow melatonin production and help you be more alert.

Use "warm" or more yellow-colored lighting closer to 3000K in color temperature in your bedroom or other areas where you spend your time in the evening. Then turn all artificial lighting *down during evening hours*. Avoiding bright and blue-toned light in the evening allows your body to produce extra melatonin and helps you sleep. Relying on natural light or simply dimming your lights late in the day (dimmers are relatively inexpensive and save electricity) will also improve your sleep quality.

Then eliminate as much light as you can in your bedroom. If you read in bed each night, use a small reading light instead of brighter overhead lighting. Add room-darkening curtains, cover any artificial light from clocks or electronic devices, and remove any other distractions. There is a reason why most hotels provide "blackout" shades for their guests. They understand that you getting a good night of sleep and being satisfied with your stay depends on keeping all light out at night.

Another good idea is to eliminate nighttime television in your bedroom. Or don't put a television in your bedroom at all. If you are used to falling asleep watching TV, try to break that habit.

○ ○ ○

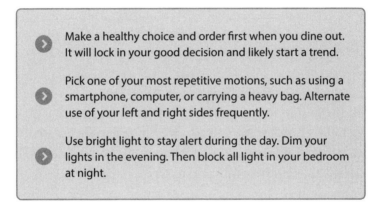

Make a healthy choice and order first when you dine out. It will lock in your good decision and likely start a trend.

Pick one of your most repetitive motions, such as using a smartphone, computer, or carrying a heavy bag. Alternate use of your left and right sides frequently.

Use bright light to stay alert during the day. Dim your lights in the evening. Then block all light in your bedroom at night.

Prioritize Your Protein

Most of us need to consume more plant-based protein and fewer carbohydrates. Research suggests protein stimulates the cells that keep us thin and alert. Yet it can be difficult to figure out how to get enough protein from the *right sources*.

In the early 2000s, like millions of other people, I jumped on the bandwagon of diets focused on added protein from *any* source. I found myself eating substantially more red meat and cheese. At the time, grilling meat each evening was easy and appealing, until I had my cholesterol checked and it had soared to a new high.

This was also the period in my life when tumors in my kidneys and pancreas grew faster than ever before. While the tumor growth could be coincidental, the way this "meat and cheese" diet increased my cholesterol was not. Fortunately, reversing the bad trend in my cholesterol levels was relatively easy as I learned about eating the right forms of protein.

Research has shown how consumption of specific protein sources can provide the nutrients you need, without the negative effects of hot dogs, hamburgers, or pastrami sandwiches. While it may be okay to eat meat occasionally, you can get all the protein you need from plant-based sources. The list below is a general continuum of where to look for protein before resorting to red or processed meats:

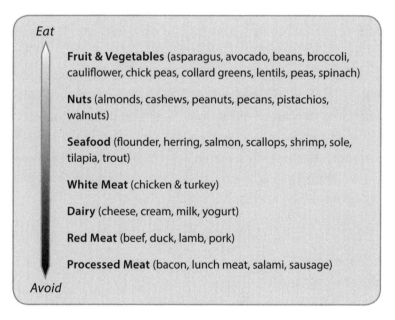

Eat

Fruit & Vegetables (asparagus, avocado, beans, broccoli, cauliflower, chick peas, collard greens, lentils, peas, spinach)

Nuts (almonds, cashews, peanuts, pecans, pistachios, walnuts)

Seafood (flounder, herring, salmon, scallops, shrimp, sole, tilapia, trout)

White Meat (chicken & turkey)

Dairy (cheese, cream, milk, yogurt)

Red Meat (beef, duck, lamb, pork)

Processed Meat (bacon, lunch meat, salami, sausage)

Avoid

Getting more protein from fruits, vegetables, nuts, and fish will also increase your intake of omega-3s, which are deficient in most people's diets today. Omega-3s are essential fatty acids shown to protect against certain cancers, cognitive decline, macular degeneration, and heart disease. They can also decrease depressive symptoms and improve your mood.

One experiment found that participants who consumed omega-3s had a 20 percent reduction in anxiety levels and a significant reduction in inflammation, compared with a control group. A 2012 study revealed that people with low levels of omega-3s even had *smaller brains* (on MRI scans) and lower scores on tests of basic mental ability. Ideal sources of omega-3s are fish, nuts, and seeds; salmon, walnuts, and flaxseeds are the best of the bunch.

Base most of your meals around protein from plant-based sources and seafood with the lowest mercury levels (as listed on the previous page). If the majority of your protein comes from these sources with higher omega-3 content, you may notice a difference in how you feel each day. Eating the right mix of these foods can boost your mood *and* improve your long-term health.

○ ○ ○

Stop Buying Junk for Friends

In the grocery store, I find it easy to rationalize buying cookies by telling myself I am "getting them for friends" or to serve at an event. So I am essentially acknowledging that a food is not healthy enough for me but still okay to give to loved ones or friends. Then I present it to my friends in a way that makes them feel good about receiving the unhealthy cookies and virtually obligate them to eat it.

What's really happening is: *I am telling others that I value their health and well-being less than my own.* Studies show that people consistently buy less healthy foods for others than for themselves. When making food purchases for themselves, people buy a balance of foods. However, when choosing food for family or friends, people are more likely to buy junk food.

As a parent of young children, I notice that almost every gathering is filled with baked goods and sweets. It is almost impossible to make a good choice at these events. When I watch sporting events with friends, the options are even more limited. I can't remember the last time I watched football with friends and ate something that was a part of my typical healthy diet.

Until I thought this through, my decisions when entertaining were as bad as anyone else's. My standard plan for having guests over was to order pizza or grill burgers. Then I realized it might be time to value the health of others as much as I value my own. Put yourself in the place of one of your friends, family members, or dinner guests. How often do you go somewhere and the food options are not as healthy or diverse as what you would select on your own?

The problem is, most of us want healthy options for ourselves but assume incorrectly that others prefer less healthy foods. Change this trend in your networks, and start bringing healthier food to gatherings. If nothing else, it will tell your friends you value their health as much as your own.

○ ○ ○

Find Your Motivation to Move

Even though people know they should exercise regularly, a majority fail to do so. We know that increasing activity levels will help us achieve major goals (e.g., losing weight) or life outcomes (e.g., living longer). But when we think about these big ultimate goals in the distance, it can be hard to get motivated today. So instead of letting these broad long-term goals overwhelm you, pick specific reasons that personally motivate you to be more active right now.

One of my best near-term motivators is better interactions with friends, colleagues, and family members. When I have been sitting all day, I get cranky — and it shows. But when I exercise early, I have more energy and a better disposition all day. There are other benefits as well: Once my workout is behind me, I feel like I have accomplished more by midday than I otherwise would in a full workday. And the vain side of me realizes my face has more color when I exercise, so I look healthier as a result.

A longer-term motivator for me is to be an active parent for many years. When I pair this motivation with my own risk factors, I have a deeply personal incentive for making good decisions. If lifestyle can prevent two-thirds of all cancers, and studies suggest exercise extends life span for those of us with cancer, it is even easier for me to make these choices. To remind myself of this each day, I keep pictures of my wife and kids directly above my desk and treadmill. This reminds me that my staying active matters as much for the people I care about as it does for myself.

Everyone has unique motivators. Some of the most powerful accounts I have heard are from people who broke the difficult habit of smoking because they knew how much it would mean to a spouse or child. Friends who have lost a lot of weight often attribute their turnaround to a deeply emotional plea from a loved one.

It is well-established that exercise reduces your risk of cancer, heart disease, high blood pressure, obesity, and depression. Activity also slows aging. There is no shortage of reasons to move more today.

◦ ◦ ◦

> Investigate how you can get most of your protein from plant-based sources.

> Quit giving people food you know better than to eat yourself. When buying food for friends or preparing a meal for others, think of what's best for their health.

> Pick one deeply personal motivation to move more. Find a way to remind yourself every day with a photo, note, or quote.

Working

Keep Work From Killing You

In 1951, a team of researchers embarked on an 18-year study of San Francisco dock workers to examine the factors that predisposed these men to fatal coronary heart disease. When they published their findings nearly two decades later, many of the usual suspects emerged as contributors to heart disease: elevated blood pressure, cigarette smoking, and obesity.

Yet one of the most striking findings was that the men with *short bursts of activity as part of their routine work* had significantly lower death rates from coronary disease. These were the dock workers who loaded cargo as new ships came in and out of port. This is the type of regular activity that was built in to a wide variety of jobs just 50 years ago.

Back then, jobs requiring moderate physical activity accounted for about half of the labor market. Today, only

20 percent of jobs require real activity. This transformational shift mirrors increases in diabetes and obesity rates. You can now accomplish countless tasks with click of a mouse and a few keystrokes. While this increases efficiency, it comes at the expense of our physical health.

This epidemic of inactivity now spans the globe. From the United States to India and China, technology — from computers to washing machines — minimizes the need for manual labor, and our health suffers as a result. The way we cook, clean, work, and make products no longer requires strenuous activity.

Because of these seismic shifts in activity levels, you now have to find ways to infuse deliberate movement into your day. If you work in a traditional office setting, it is in your company's best interest to ensure you get some activity during the workday.

Emerging research suggests companies that provide employees with time to exercise, even during working hours, do not lose any business. In fact, this research shows how you could be *more productive* if your organization gives you time to exercise *during the workday*. Even when you work fewer hours in a week, the tradeoff is a net positive for you and your organization. Other studies find that employees see significant increases in overall earnings as their activity levels rise.

The good news is, many employers are taking notice. A friend of mine recently lost 50 pounds. When I asked him how he did it, he gave almost all the credit to encouragement from his colleagues and programs his employer offered. Even if your peer group at work is not very active, consider what you can do to start a positive trend.

Find a few moments each day when you can walk briskly. Do a few push-ups or anything else to break up a 10-hour span of limited activity. Ask a colleague to go for a walking meeting instead of sitting in uncomfortable chairs. The late Steve Jobs was famous for requiring colleagues and clients to go on walking meetings around his neighborhood. When a reporter asked him why he did, Jobs explained he could think better when he walked.

If nothing else, make sure you get up several times a day and move around your workspace. Work can make you fat, sick, and tired. But building movement into your daily routine will provide a buffer against today's sedentary jobs. As a leading public health researcher put it, "In many ways we've engineered physical activity out of our lives, so we've got to find ways to put it back into our lives."

◉ ◉ ◉

The Danger of Desktop Dining

Early in my career, having lunch with a group of friends from work was one of the best parts of my day. Some days we would all go out to eat, but most of the time, we grabbed lunch in the cafeteria. Either way, it provided a mental break from what I was working on and forced me to get up and move around. Most importantly, it was quality social time with my friends.

However, as the demands of my job increased over the next couple of years, my lunchtime pattern changed. On most days, I considered myself too busy for an extended lunch and opted to eat at my desk. This allowed me to devour my food as quickly as possible, usually hunched over my keyboard reading email. Eating at my desk got lunch "out of the way" in about five minutes, compared to the 50 minutes it took to eat with a group.

I justified eating at my desk by telling myself it made me more productive. In hindsight, desktop dining had the opposite effect. It was bad for my relationships with colleagues. I had less physical energy. And I was less satisfied with my job at the end of the workday and had fewer ideas to contribute.

When I have a busy day, I still eat at my desk more than I should. But I can now see how it is a trap because I eat more at my desk than I do when I am paying attention. By sitting and eating at my desk, I also miss an opportunity for midday activity.

According to various studies, roughly two-thirds of workers eat lunch at their desks. And a majority don't take time for regular breaks during the workday. This can result in trouble focusing and less time for creative thought. So to prevent that, use lunch as a natural stopping point in the middle of a busy day. Take a short walk. On nice days, get outside for fresh air. Or find somewhere to eat with a few friends at work. Use lunchtime as a reminder to get exercise and energizing social time.

○ ○ ○

Working While Intoxicated

Sleep less, achieve less. It's really that simple. According to a study from Harvard Medical School, lack of sleep costs the American economy $63 billion a year in lost productivity alone. In the words of one of the lead researchers, "Americans are not missing work because of insomnia. They are still going to their jobs but they're accomplishing less because they're tired. In an information-based economy, it's difficult to find a condition that has a greater effect on productivity."

Sleep-deprived driving can be as hazardous as drunk driving; 75 percent of the time a truck driver runs someone off the road, driver fatigue is a prominent factor. According to one scientist who has studied this extensively, four hours of sleep loss produces as much impairment as a six-pack of beer. A whole night of sleep loss is equivalent to a staggering blood alcohol level of 0.19 percent. That's double most legal limits.

Working on little sleep is not much better. There is a reason why surgeons and pilots now have mandated periods of rest before they are allowed to operate or fly an airplane. In 2010, an Air India 737 crashed, killing 158 people. When investigators listened to the data recorder, what they heard was "heavy nasal snoring" in the cockpit. This is just one example; hundreds are killed every year by people who get too little sleep.

If you care about the quality of your work and interactions with your peers, give sleep the priority it deserves. To make this possible, your work needs to be satisfying. Poor sleep quality is nearly twice as common among those who are least satisfied with their jobs.

Even if you are not in your dream job today, it's up to you to make sure work is not keeping you up every night. Any job is likely to cause a sleepless night on occasion. But I'm amazed by how many people go through weeks, months, or years of dealing with poor sleep due to job stress. It's hard to imagine that any job is worth the damage this does to your health over time.

○ ○ ○

> Engineer activity into your work. Have a standing or walking meeting. Get up and move every time you are on the phone.

> Take a midday break of at least 30 minutes every day.

> Structure your work schedule for better sleep. Help your boss and colleagues understand why good sleep is in everyone's best interest.

Quitting

The Throwaway Foods

Some foods have no redeeming value for anyone. Yet the first thing people do when they receive a big box of candy they don't want is put it in a common location for others to consume. Who will pass on free food, right?

A couple of years ago, I spoke to a group of leaders about the importance of wellness in the workplace. Following my talk, I received a giant bucket of candy from the event's organizers as a thank you. I'm sure they had the best intentions, but it was ironic, given the topic I covered. Nonetheless, when I got back to my office, I scoured through the bucket in search of anything remotely healthy. No luck. Out of 20 options, they were all loaded with sugar and refined carbohydrates.

To keep myself from eating these sweets, I would normally put the bucket in our office's shared kitchen or offer the candy to someone else. But as I thought about it, that decision made little sense. If I left the bucket in our office kitchen, my friends and colleagues would walk by, be tempted to take some, and be less healthy as a result.

Given that more than one-third of our sugar intake comes from snacks, leaving this candy out for colleagues suddenly felt like the wrong decision. If I care about the people I work with, why tempt them to make a lousy choice? So I dumped the entire bucket of sweets into a garbage can in my office. *Many foods are better off in the trash than in your stomach.*

The next time you receive unhealthy food as a gift, subtly dispose of it later. When you get a free dessert or candy with a meal, leave it behind. If the item is clearly bad for your health, don't feel guilty. You are not wasting food. You may be saving lives.

○ ○ ○

Help a Quitter Win

When you pass on a piece of cake, it inevitably leads to someone saying, "Come on, one bite won't kill you." Loved ones, friends, and colleagues say this all the time. They do it without much thought or any bad intentions.

Yet for those who are trying to eat well and avoid sugary desserts, these innocent comments make it difficult to resist temptation. While it is common to pressure someone to take one bite of cake, you know better than to tell a friend who is an alcoholic he should just have one drink.

People with drug or alcohol addictions can stay away from bars or environments that create temptation. However, those who are diabetic or obese do not have the option to completely avoid food. So making good dietary decisions will be a daily struggle for the rest of their lives.

Our social circles continue to make this even more difficult. Half of people surveyed in one study reported feeling pressure from peers to eat foods that are not on their diet; 35 percent reported that other people go as far as to make jokes about their diet. Nearly one-third said that someone had *ordered food for them* at a restaurant they would not have selected for dietary reasons.

Then you have the subtle social pressures that cause us to make poor decisions; 56 percent of people in this survey broke their diet to avoid insulting a host, boss, client, or family member. Another 51 percent did so because they wanted to eat like everyone else and fit in with the group.

Instead of doing things that unintentionally sabotage the health of others, turn this social influence in the other direction. Acknowledge friends who decide to pass on cake or ice cream for the sake of their health. Give them credit in front of the group, or better yet, join them in making healthy decisions.

Try quitting a few of the worst foods you eat. Set a good example with your own choices in social settings. You don't have to be one of those obnoxious people at a dinner, espousing your dietary beliefs to anyone who will listen. Instead, help friends understand your decisions if they ask. Once you quit ordering cake, you will notice friends doing the same over time, even if it never comes up in conversation.

● ● ●

Hit Snooze and You Lose

The snooze button seems so innocent. For decades, it was a close friend of mine. It was rare if a day went by when I did not give myself an extra 15 minutes of sleep after the alarm rang. And for many people, the snooze button ritual lasts for 30-60 minutes. This might be fine if we weren't already struggling to get enough sound sleep.

When you break your final hour of sleep into small half-awake chunks, studies show *it does not count* toward the total amount of deep restorative sleep. For the next few weeks, set your alarm at the latest possible time so hitting the snooze button is not an option. Force yourself to get up right away. Those extra minutes can give you enough sleep so you feel refreshed.

If promising not to hit snooze doesn't work, move your alarm clock beyond your reach so you have to get out of bed to turn off the alarm. Find a clock or smartphone app designed to prevent you from snoozing. Or if all else fails, get one of those clocks that automatically rolls off your nightstand and forces you to chase it across the room.

If you naturally wake up at around the same time each day, another option is to do away with your alarm altogether — though this might not be practical if your job requires an early start. One friend of mine banished the alarm clock from his bedroom. After waking up without using an alarm clock for several years, he describes how peaceful his mornings are compared with the days when he was awakened by a jarring noise.

The light from an alarm clock can also be an issue. If the display on your clock is one of the brightest elements in your bedroom, you are likely to glance at it when you are having trouble sleeping. When you look over and see you're still awake at 2 a.m., all it does is create even more stress and keep you up longer.

A simple solution I found is a clock that requires me to push a button on top if I need to see the time. It does not display the time continuously in an otherwise dark room. When I am in a hotel, I make sure to turn the alarm clock around or cover the display. These small changes helped far more than I would have guessed.

● ● ●

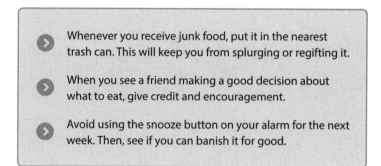

> Whenever you receive junk food, put it in the nearest trash can. This will keep you from splurging or regifting it.

> When you see a friend making a good decision about what to eat, give credit and encouragement.

> Avoid using the snooze button on your alarm for the next week. Then, see if you can banish it for good.

The Butter Is Healthier Than the Bread

When I was growing up, I was told that anything made with wheat was good for me. As it turns out, a couple pieces of bread could increase blood sugar as much as a can of sugary soda or a candy bar. The original study that launched the concept of the glycemic index (GI) as a measure of the effects of certain foods on our blood sugar revealed that the GI of whole grain bread is 72 (lower number is better). For comparison, the GI for white bread is 69, a Mars candy bar is 68, shredded wheat cereal is 67, and table sugar is 59. A more recent study found that foods containing the industry standard "whole grain stamp" were *higher* in sugar and calories than products without the stamp.

Surrounding a healthy food with two slices of bread changes the entire equation. According to one expert, eating two pieces of whole wheat bread increases your blood sugar *more than eating two tablespoons of pure sugar*. This triggers the release of insulin and eventually leads to the growth of extra abdominal fat. As this cycle continues, higher blood sugar levels signal an inflammatory response, increasing the odds of bigger problems like heart disease and cancer.

Do all you can to eat less bread. Take the top slice off a sandwich so you consume half as much. Better yet, replace bread with a bed of greens for a much healthier option.

Many "healthy" menu options at restaurants, from fast food to dine-in, include a roll or bread on the side. This is the default for most restaurants, and it is what consumers expect. My three favorite lunch spots provide bread with each salad. The amount of bread they include is about the same portion size you get with a sandwich. So, if I were to eat the bread, it defeats the purpose of getting a salad instead of a sandwich.

Every day at these restaurants, I see people who, with great intentions, order a relatively healthy salad but also take the free bread. The vast majority take the bread, which means they also eat these additional carbs and calories. My favorite entrée salad, for example, has 16 grams of carbohydrates. The supposedly healthy "whole grain flatbread" they include for free (which makes it even harder to decline) adds a whopping 46 grams of carbs. The bread nearly triples the total carbohydrates for this meal.

The obvious, but admittedly difficult, choice is to turn down the side of bread. Then you don't need to worry about the temptation or the guilt of throwing food away. Or request a substitute for the bread, like carrots or apples. I have been pleasantly surprised by how many restaurants will provide a much healthier alternative if you ask.

There will always be times when you are eating on the run and a wrap or sandwich is the only viable option. The key is to pass on all of the extra bread. As one of the world's leading researchers on obesity put it, the next time you consume buttered toast, consider that the butter may be healthier than the bread.

◎ ◎ ◎

Don't Eat Your Meat and Potatoes

Meat and potatoes are central to a Western diet. Growing up in Nebraska, an agricultural state in the middle of the U.S., my two dietary staples were meat and some form of potato. Like most of my peers, as a child, I was told to eat my meat and potatoes if I wanted to grow up to be big, strong, and healthy. According to the research, I was not alone in associating meat with masculinity.

However, these two foods are at the root of a global obesity epidemic. A large-scale study published in the *New England Journal of Medicine* revealed that french fries and potato chips account for even more weight gain over time than processed and red meat. This study suggests that the combination of these "meat and potato" categories could add more pounds to your waistline than sweets and desserts.

While a moderate amount of meat and potato products may not be a problem, watch out for excessive quantities of these two foods in particular. Research suggests that eating processed meat regularly (e.g., sausage or bacon) can increase the risk of deadly pancreatic cancer by 19 percent for men. This is one of several studies to identify an association between higher meat consumption and long-term health problems.

The most comprehensive study of its kind, which followed more than 100,000 men and women over 28 years, found that one daily serving of processed red meat (e.g., one hot dog or two slices of bacon) was associated with a 20 percent increased risk of death during the study period. One serving a day was also linked to a 21 percent higher risk of dying from heart disease and a 16 percent higher risk of dying from cancer. Similar but slightly smaller risk levels were found for unprocessed meat. These studies suggest that *daily consumption* of red and processed meat, in particular, poses the highest risk.

Start thinking about what you could substitute for meat and potatoes. For example, replace one serving of processed meat with vegetables, fish, nuts, or legumes. It might be unrealistic to eliminate these two staples from your diet entirely, so try to cut back by making meat and potatoes something you consume only occasionally.

Be Cold in Bed

It is easier to sleep in a dark, cool room than in a warm room. You have a natural body clock that regulates your core temperature, and fluctuations tell you when to sleep and when to wake. If a room is too warm, your body clock will think it is time to wake up, regardless of the time. This explains why you can fall asleep easier and sleep longer in a cool room.

Experts advise keeping your thermostat two to four degrees cooler at night. This is not ideal if you live where the climate makes cooling an entire home to this range less energy efficient. Some things you can do to help include: opening and closing vents to keep your bedroom cooler than the rest of the house, installing a secondary thermostat to maintain a cooler temperature in the bedroom, using lighter or fewer blankets, running a fan at night, or adding a gel-based mattress topper to keep your bed cool at night.

Try to sleep in a room that is a few degrees cooler than the temperature you are accustomed to during the day. This mild drop in temperature induces sleep. As part of one experiment, researchers had insomniacs wear "cooling caps" and found that this alternative was three times as effective at helping them sleep as sleeping pills. Other research goes as far as to suggest that rising indoor temperatures could be contributing to obesity. Turning the thermostat down could even help you shed a few pounds.

At a minimum, a slightly cooler room can help you get a good night's sleep. Another thing to remember is *all sleep temperatures are relative* to what your body is accustomed to during the day. In the summer, for example, I sleep with a warmer bedroom temperature (73 degrees) than I do during the winter (68 degrees) to conserve energy. What matters is that the temperature is two to four degrees cooler than what you are accustomed to during the day, whether it is summer or winter.

○ ○ ○

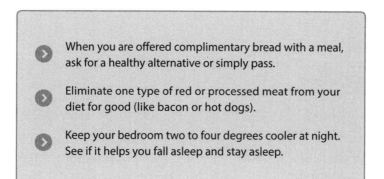

> When you are offered complimentary bread with a meal, ask for a healthy alternative or simply pass.

> Eliminate one type of red or processed meat from your diet for good (like bacon or hot dogs).

> Keep your bedroom two to four degrees cooler at night. See if it helps you fall asleep and stay asleep.

Home

Small Plates, Smaller Waistline

Portion sizes in most homes and restaurants today are larger than necessary. Unfortunately, we often rely on a visual scan of our plates, instead of our stomach, to determine when we are full. Studies show that when we have a larger portion size, we eat substantially more food.

A set of experiments revealed how poorly the internal fuel gauge on your stomach functions. When you are given an extra-large container of popcorn, you eat 45 percent more. You pour 37 percent more liquid in short and wide cups compared with tall and skinny cups. The effect was even worse for kids, who served themselves *twice as much cereal* if given a 16-ounce bowl instead of an 8-ounce bowl.

When preparing your next few meals at home, use smaller plates like those intended for side salads or appetizers. After trying this for several months, I found that these plates, which are 30-50 percent smaller in total area, are enough to hold the amount of food I need. Until I did the math, I did not realize a traditional 11-inch plate has nearly *double* the surface area (95 square inches) of an 8-inch plate (50 square inches).

Use plates with a diameter closer to the length of your hand than to the length of your foot. If you do not have smaller plates, try to place smaller total portions on your larger plates. Start by placing food at the center of the plate instead of circling the edges. The goal is not to fill every inch of space on your plate with food.

Even the color of a plate can influence what you eat. A study published in the *Journal of Consumer Research* suggests that the impact of plate color alone is quite dramatic. They found a clear *contrast between food and plate* keeps people from overeating. In the experiments, for example, when pasta with white sauce was served on a white plate, people consumed nearly 30 percent more pasta compared with those who received the same meal on a red plate.

Be even more conscious about how much you eat when the color of your food matches the color of your plate. White is the most common plate color, and white-colored foods are often the least healthy. Consider all the foods that blend into a white background, from pasta to white bread to mashed potatoes. These are foods you should try to avoid, yet a matching white plate color can trick you into eating more of these foods.

Of course, I'm not suggesting you go out and buy green plates tomorrow so you can eat loads of broccoli with less effort. But pay extra attention to how much food you put on your plate, especially when it blends into the background. If you use white plates, add contrast to each meal with healthy reds, greens, and darker colored foods.

● ● ●

Staying Active Starts at Home

If you want change to last, start at home. A study of more than 6,000 people who had been successful keeping weight off revealed that the most effective and sustainable changes start in the home. Ninety-two percent of the participants in this study found a way to exercise in their homes. Whether you use a treadmill, elliptical machine, stair stepper, or video-based aerobic program or exercise out in your neighborhood, your home is a great place to build an active lifestyle.

This study also revealed that 78 percent of the participants ate breakfast every day, which is much easier to do if you establish a routine at home. Another 75 percent of the most successful group weighed themselves once a week. The fourth most common habit, identified by two-thirds of people in this study, was watching less than 10 hours of television per week.

As you can see from the common threads of those who successfully kept weight off, most of these habits revolve around what goes on at home. This is where we construct our daily defaults, for better or worse. When you want to establish a new routine that benefits your health, start with what goes on where you live.

Finding excuses for *not* exercising is easy. Making the decision *to* exercise is not. I have trouble just getting out of bed early enough to work out. If this is as big a challenge for you as it is for me, eliminate little things that get in your way each morning.

Start with a few small adjustments. Set your workout gear next to your bed at night so you barely have to get up to get rolling. If you drink coffee, set your coffee maker on a timer so you wake up to the smell of freshly brewed coffee. If going to the gym is an obstacle, build your routine around an at-home workout. Turn activity into the path of least resistance.

○ ○ ○

Make Sleep a Family Value

Sleep is a treasure, and it should be valued as one. Yet for many of us, sleep is the first thing we cast aside. In my own experience growing up, I recall several of my role models boasting about running on just a few hours of sleep.

In hindsight, I know that this was rooted in a good-natured work ethic. Yet my major takeaway at a young age was that needing a lot of sleep was a sign of weakness. This made it easier for me to spend my teenage years up late at night, doing absolutely nothing productive.

Today, researchers have identified a strong link between children's sleep patterns and their performance in the classroom. They found simply having a specific bedtime rule makes a profound difference. Children with higher sleep quality are more active and eat healthier foods. All of this research suggests we need to rethink sleep as a core family value.

Help the people you live with understand and appreciate that sleep is beneficial for everyone. If you have children, don't send them to bed as punishment. Think about the message it sends. And set a good example by consistently getting quality sleep yourself.

A good friend of mine whose children are now in high school described how their family has maintained sleep as a core value for a couple of decades. They always put their kids to bed early, starting at a young age, and allowed them to read as long as they wanted. Even now that their kids are older, they have no computers or televisions in their bedrooms. Every night, they still read before bed, and the entire family sleeps well. This is just one example of how to build a healthy routine for kids, but it is likely to work for us adults as well.

Consider how you can help spouses, friends, and roommates sleep better. Make a goal of helping everyone under your roof get sound sleep. Talk about how schedules, lights, thermostats, and noise can be adjusted to help everyone sleep. It is clearly in your best interest to ensure the people you spend time with are well-rested. No one likes perpetually grumpy housemates.

○ ○ ○

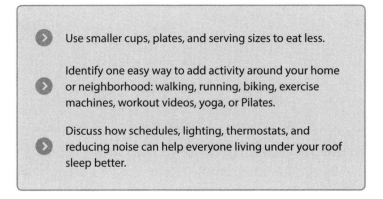

> Use smaller cups, plates, and serving sizes to eat less.

> Identify one easy way to add activity around your home or neighborhood: walking, running, biking, exercise machines, workout videos, yoga, or Pilates.

> Discuss how schedules, lighting, thermostats, and reducing noise can help everyone living under your roof sleep better.

Get Ahead

Don't Be Fooled by the Decoy

Restaurants know how to lure us in. They have sophisticated research showing how placing salads and other healthy options on the menu — *even if we don't buy them* — allows us to justify going there in the first place. We are more likely to visit a less healthy restaurant *when a healthy option is available* compared with when no healthy options are available. It is hard to believe how well this works. A less healthy restaurant plants a healthy decoy, and it gives us an excuse to dine there.

I fell into this trap myself recently. While driving and growing increasingly hungry, I noticed a national burger chain that had been running ad campaigns touting their new "garden salads." To justify pulling off the road,

I told myself I would order the salad. However, by the time I reached the drive-through window, some irrational impulse made me order a cheeseburger and fries instead. Restaurants know we make these crazy justifications and use it against us. *Before you even decide on a restaurant* with one of your favorite indulgent choices, remember it is a game you will likely lose.

When you eat at a chain restaurant, making good choices is even more challenging. A massive U.S. Department of Agriculture study, which examined the nutritional content of 30,923 menu items from 245 popular restaurant brands, uncovered a widespread problem. Among top restaurant chains in this study, 97 percent of entrées exceeded daily limits for calories, sodium, and saturated fat.

This does not mean you need to abandon dining out. Getting out with friends and family is, of course, a good idea for a host of other reasons. What it means is you have to be even more selective about where you go and what you order. Find a restaurant with several healthy options on the menu that are as appealing as indulgent choices. This will make it easier to dine there regularly, select from a range of foods, and eat relatively healthy.

Start with the right place to eat. If you wind up at a restaurant with limited options, do your best to play defense. Ask for your sandwich without mayonnaise. To make sure your salad is not soaked in high-calorie dressing, ask for light dressing, or better yet, get it on the side.

Skip the bacon on a burger. Ask for steamed vegetables instead of veggies sautéed in butter or covered with cheese. Avoid deep-fried options. Slowly chip away at bad habits to make better choices.

◎ ◎ ◎

Structure Exercise for Enjoyment

The hardest part of working out for me is the first five minutes. I know if I am going to run outdoors, as long as I *start*, I am likely to keep going. The same goes for cold days when I exercise on my elliptical machine. If I'm not feeling up to working out on a particular day, I tell myself I only need to exercise for 10 minutes. Then by that point, I usually feel great and keep going for at least 30 minutes. It's all mental trickery, but it works.

No matter how much you care about your health, there is a good chance you still dread your daily workout, at least some of the time. Most of us underestimate the enjoyment value of exercise — from group workouts, individual exercise, moderate activity, challenging workouts, and everything from yoga to weight training. Apparently the *thought* of exercise, at least when you consider it in advance, is a deterrent.

The good news is, we enjoy exercise more in the moment (e.g., when we're running or in a yoga class) than we estimate in advance. According to researchers who studied this phenomenon extensively, one reason we underestimate enjoyment is because we place *too much focus* on the often unpleasant *beginning* of the activity. If you reflect on a recent workout, it is likely you experienced a peak moment in the middle of the event and felt pretty good at the end of your workout as well.

Several studies show that people tend to remember the *peaks* and *ends* of any experience. So try to focus on a peak moment during your last workout, perhaps when you had a real rush of energy. Also consider the sense of gratification you had when you finished.

If you structure your activity to end on a high note, you are more likely to do it again. As part of an experiment on this topic, participants were assigned to exercise for 20 minutes at a level they considered unpleasant. In one of the sessions, they had a pleasant five-minute cool-down period added to the end of the workout. In another session, there was no cool down. When researchers asked participants which workout they would repeat a week later, they chose the one with the pleasant end by a ratio of 2 to 1.

Another strategy to coax yourself into exercising is to select the part of your routine you enjoy most and move it up to the beginning of your workout. Anything that makes it easier for you to get started instead of postponing exercise helps. Find some way to focus on the easiest and most enjoyable parts of your workout, and then close it out on a good note.

A Night to Remember

While it seems obvious that good sleep provides extra brainpower for the next day, you may underestimate how sleep influences your ability to make sense of what you learned *the day before*. In the span of a full day, you take in large amounts of disparate information. With all the input your brain needs to process in a day, it is no wonder some form of memory consolidation must occur. You simply cannot retain everything.

This is when a sound night's sleep comes into play. It helps your mind work through an unconscious process. While you are asleep, your brain goes back through the day's events and selects the most pertinent knowledge. These key memories are then reinforced and encoded for long-term storage. This is what allows you to recall certain facts or events later.

Think back to when you were a student. Someone likely told you to get a good night's sleep and to eat a healthy breakfast before a test or final exam. The theory is, you need to be fresh to perform well.

However, while getting sound sleep the night before a test is a good idea, it is too late to help you on the test. The real benefit comes from getting good sleep as you learn throughout the year, so the information can be encoded in your memory each night. If you file everything away properly as you go along, this knowledge will be there for you when you need it most.

This is more than an interesting theory. It has been tested in several experimental settings. These studies show how sleep duration and quality aid your ability to recall specific facts you learned the day *before*. Research also suggests that chronic sleep impairment is bad for your overall mental ability and akin to aging four to seven years. If you sleep well, it essentially keeps your mental hard drive from failing.

○ ○ ○

> Select restaurants based on how easy it is to make a healthy choice when you order.

> When you are tempted to skip a workout, just start exercising for a few minutes. Starting is often the hardest part.

> The next time you work on something that requires a great deal of learning and synthesizing, go to bed early instead of staying up late.

Energy

Avoid a High-Fat Hangover

While I was in the middle of working on this book, my
mom called on a beautiful fall weekend and asked if she
could take our family out for Sunday brunch. She had
picked a nearby restaurant that was getting great reviews.
When we got there, it was bustling with people and an
enthusiastic staff. But when I scanned the limited brunch
menu, I realized it was going to be difficult to make a
good choice.

There were just five options on the menu. None of
them looked particularly healthy. When our server intro-
duced herself, she described how the glazed doughnuts
with chocolate sauce and eggs Benedict were the two most
popular items. I ordered the eggs Benedict, figuring it was

not as bad as the doughnuts and telling myself I deserved a "cheat day." When my meal arrived, the English muffin with ham and two poached eggs smothered in a thick hollandaise sauce was accompanied by a buttery biscuit and fried potatoes, which I ate as well.

We had a great time at the restaurant, and the meal was filled with good flavors. However, by early afternoon, I was bloated and half asleep on my couch. It was one of the nicest days of the year and my daughter was asking me to take her to the nearby park, but my energy was zapped. For the rest of the day, my high-fat hangover from that one meal prevented me from doing anything enjoyable or productive.

In hindsight, the only one I was cheating by making a bad breakfast decision was myself. It was a self-inflicted way to ruin my energy and well-being for the remainder of the day. A few weeks later, I was in a similar situation. This time, I made a different choice and requested a healthy item not on the menu: an egg white omelet with spinach, mushrooms, and tomatoes. That afternoon, I had all the energy in the world, played with my kids, got a little work done, and went for a run.

It is easy to take for granted how specific foods influence your energy and mood during a typical day. Yet when scientists explore the relationship between diet and mental health, it is clear that *certain types of food increase or decrease your energy* in a given day. Fatty foods, for example, can make you lethargic and moody.

One experiment found that people who consume more trans fatty acids have significantly greater levels of aggression. They are also more irritable. These findings led one of the researchers to suggest that institutions, like schools and prisons, should reconsider serving fatty foods because the detrimental impact "may extend beyond the person who consumes them to affect others."

The consumption of trans and saturated fats over time has also been shown to increase the risk of being diagnosed with depression by up to 48 percent. Eating fast food and baked goods results in similar increases in the risk of depression, even when consumed in small doses. These "comfort foods" do not provide any comfort after all and could even accelerate the cycle of depression. If you crave unhealthy foods when you are stressed, try to avoid the trap of eating them. Eating poorly will make a bad day even worse.

If you want to get your day off to a good start, don't have biscuits and gravy for breakfast. Before you order a heavy lunch, think about whether you can afford what one scientist dubbed a "high-fat hangover." Consider the possibility, as researchers are investigating, that unhealthy food for dinner can increase tensions with your spouse.

Each time you decide what to eat, it subtly shapes your days and interactions with others. Fortunately, eating the right foods can turn your mood in the right direction. Research suggests that on days when you eat more fruits and vegetables, you will feel calmer, happier, and more energetic than normal.

◉ ◉ ◉

Take Your Brain for a Walk

Your brain works better following exercise. A team of researchers in Ireland made this discovery through a relatively simple experiment. They asked a group of students to watch a rapid lineup of photos. Each photo included a name and face of a stranger. Then, after a brief break, the students tried to recall the names of the faces that had moved across the computer screen. After this initial test, half of the students were asked to ride a stationary bicycle at a strenuous pace until they reached exhaustion. The other half of the students sat quietly for 30 minutes. Then both groups took the test again to see how many names they could recall.

The group of students who exercised performed much better on the memory test than they had on their first attempt. The group who simply sat in another room did not improve. As part of this experiment, the scientists also collected blood samples, through which they discovered a biological explanation for the increase in recall among the students who exercised. Immediately after the strenuous activity, students in the exercise group had much higher levels of a protein known as brain-derived neurotrophic factor, or BDNF, which promotes the health of nerve cells.

Based on this research and other emerging experiments, exercise creates an immediate benefit for your memory. Once your brain initially processes something, you are less likely to retain the information if you are not physically active in the period following this learning. If you *learn then move*, you will have more effective recall when you need it most.

Walking a mile a day at least six days a week can even keep your brain from shrinking. As part of an ongoing 20-year longitudinal study, researchers analyzed the relationship between activity levels and brain structure in more than 400 people. These scientists monitored how far people walked each week. Then all patients underwent 3D MRI scans to identify changes in brain volume. When brain volume decreases, it suggests cells are dying.

This study revealed that higher levels of physical activity are consistently related to greater brain volume. For healthy adults in the study without any signs of cognitive impairment, walking about a mile a day was enough to maintain brain volume. It also significantly reduced their risk for cognitive decline. Other studies have shown that similar levels of activity could reduce the risk of early death by at least 20 percent.

In addition to all the obvious benefits of walking, such as giving you a quick mental refresher and energy, it is also essential for maintaining your cognitive ability as you age. To fuel creativity now and prevent memory loss over time, get walking.

Try Exercise Instead of Sleeping Pills

Regular exercise may be the best way to ensure a good night's sleep and more energy the following day. In particular, if you are among the 35 to 40 percent who have trouble falling asleep or who get tired during the day, vigorous activity is a better place to start than medication. As sleep researcher Brad Cardinal put it, "The scientific evidence is encouraging as regular physical activity may serve as a non-pharmaceutical alternative to improve sleep."

Cardinal's research team found, after controlling for known risk factors, that sleeplessness decreased by 65 percent for participants who met the basic activity guideline of 150 minutes of exercise per week. People who worked out regularly also had less difficulty concentrating during the day. Another researcher on this team said, "Regular physical activity may positively influence an individual's productivity at work, or in the case of the student, influence their ability to pay attention in class."

If you want better sleep, even a workout late in the day beats no exercise at all. While working out early can boost your mood for the day, *late-day activity is just as valuable for your sleep*. Despite what you might have heard about exercise at night disrupting sleep, studies on this topic show that even vigorous workouts in the hours right before bed are likely to *improve* sleep significantly.

It's easy to skip your workout when you are busy, but these studies show that you are better off making sure you get some activity. Try exercising to break a long-term cycle of sleeplessness before you jump to over-the-counter or prescription sleeping medications. As is the case with a variety of common ailments, a bit of activity can be more effective than a pill.

○ ○ ○

> Before you order a heavy lunch, consider whether you can afford the hangover that afternoon.

> When your brain is filled with new information to remember or when you need a burst of creativity, go for a walk.

> If you're having trouble sleeping, try exercising for a few days before you resort to sleep medication.

Stigmatize Sinful Foods

Depending on how old you are, you might remember when it was acceptable to light up a cigarette on an airplane, in a classroom, or at your desk. But over time, smoking indoors has become socially unacceptable. The same thing occurred with littering, which was once commonplace but is now rare and illegal. More recently, you can see how similar changes in social expectations influence recycling.

I admit I didn't start recycling at home until I realized all of my neighbors were, and I felt social pressure. At my office, I used to grab paper cups for coffee every day and throw them out without thinking twice. Then, as I noticed my coworkers using reusable mugs and watching with a hint of contempt when I threw away paper cups,

I too switched to a reusable mug. My social networks discouraged my bad habits, and it led to positive change.

These same social pressures are now being aimed at unhealthy foods. I recently noticed a large sign on the window of a major fast-food chain that was featuring a sandwich. It consisted of cheese, bacon, and mayonnaise surrounded by two large pieces of *fried chicken in place of the bun*. The sign read, "We double dare you" above a photo of the sandwich. My reaction was surprise and disgust. Even if consumers are willing to buy this heart-attack-inducing sandwich, it seemed almost unconscionable for the restaurant to explicitly dare people to make a poor decision.

We can use negative social stigmas to our advantage if we start to view fatty, fried, and sugary foods with contempt. Vilifying people who are obese would clearly be a mistake, but why not *stigmatize the foods* that cause obesity, diabetes, and cancer? If you eat something regularly that you know is not good for you, give it some kind of label to create a barrier to you eating it. For example, around our house, we started calling lollipops "sugar on a stick." We described donuts as "deep-fried dough." If you make a few of your unhealthy choices less socially acceptable for yourself, it will influence the environment around you as well.

Changing the way you look at bad foods subtly improves your default choices. Learning more about the content of what I eat, versus relying on the branding, improved my dietary norms dramatically over the last decade. For example, I replaced crackers with almonds and swapped potato chips for carrots. Now when I get hungry, I reach for the healthier options as a default. Once you reset your norms and have healthy alternatives at your disposal, it is a lot easier to make good choices.

To minimize temptation, set the right dietary defaults to maximize your willpower. Researchers found that people who exhibit the most self-control are the ones who set themselves up to use their willpower the least over the course of a typical day. Every good decision you make in advance essentially makes the next few choices even easier. Instead of fighting one desire after another, set up your day to minimize temptation.

Find a few new defaults for unhealthy items you consume regularly. Identify a healthier drink to keep on hand. Think about a few of the healthiest snacks you eat. How could they substitute for things you reach for in weaker moments? As you start to build new habits around these defaults, you will notice how much less willpower it requires to get through the day.

○ ○ ○

Organic Does Not Equal Healthy

Don't confuse *organic* with *healthy*. An "organic" label on a product simply means it was grown naturally, free of pesticides, fertilizers, solvents, and chemical additives. Organic foods are essentially grown as they were in generations past, before the development of modern chemicals and additives. Back then, it was simply called food, without the need for additional distinctions.

Organic food producers attempt to eliminate chemicals, not calories. Unfortunately, many consumers gloss over this distinction and believe that organic products have lower fat, calorie, and sugar content. "Fair trade" foods fall in the same category. One study revealed that people believed the fair trade chocolate they were consuming had fewer calories.

Countless products have earned a certified organic label, yet they are filled with sugar, carbohydrates, or fats that are bad for your health. A friend once tried to convince me a dish was healthy because it was made with "organic brown sugar." Less damaging? Possibly. Healthy? No. Organic or not, sugar has a wide range of negative effects and is not good for your health. Yet experiments show that people mistakenly believe products like cookies and potato chips labeled as organic are healthier. They are also willing to pay up to 23 percent more for these unhealthy items if they have an organic label.

On packaged foods and drinks, there is usually a box on the side or back of the item that contains the most objective information about what is in the product. Study a product's full nutritional label. Carefully examine the relative levels of fats, carbs, sugars, and protein. Look at the list of ingredients to better understand the contents of the foods and drinks you are planning to consume. Compare these numbers to a few alternatives on the shelf. As you learn more about what goes into a food or drink, it can improve the quality of your choices.

Don't get me wrong. It does pay to buy organic food in some cases, but organic is far from an assurance of overall nutritional value. When you buy produce and *eat the outer layer or skin* in particular, such as berries or apples, it makes sense to select organic over conventional. But before you consider whether to buy organic, ask if the product is good for your health first. Then, figure out if it is worth buying the organic version.

● ● ●

Go Public With a Goal

To achieve a goal, share it with someone who cares. Over the last few years, I have watched several good friends use this strategy to their advantage. One friend emailed a group of her closest friends to tell them she was planning to run a half-marathon. She announced it six months in advance, which helped her to stay on track with her training.

She knew that once she put it out there, she would follow through. It worked. Another friend posted his goal of completing a triathlon on Facebook. That worked as well. What's more, both of them inspired others to join in their respective efforts.

A study published in the journal *Obesity* revealed just how contagious success is when trying to lose weight. The study found that people who were on teams with more social influence increased their odds of losing weight by 20 percent. These results show how helpful it can be to surround yourself with people who have similar health goals.

Using functional MRI scans, researchers also discovered that the brain places more value on winning when you're in a social setting than it does when you are alone. If you have a specific goal, such as running a 5K race, share your goal with a close friend. Better yet, share your goal with an entire group of friends to up the ante.

The act of sharing a goal, in itself, is likely to help. While some people are self-motivated and do not need external pressure, for most of us, it helps to create some social expectations around any major goal. Sharing your goal might even inspire the people you care about to make similar changes in their lives.

◦ ◦ ◦

> Pick one food you eat even though you know you shouldn't. Give it an entertaining nickname that will make you think twice about eating it.

> Shop for foods based on whether they are good for you first. Then consider buying organic if you eat the skin.

> Identify a specific goal for increasing your activity. Write it down, add a deadline, and share it with at least one person (ideally more) or post it online.

Good Nights

Feast at Sunrise, Fast at Sunset

Instead of skipping breakfast, make it the most important meal of your day. When you skip breakfast altogether, you are likely to eat more by the end of the day. Regularly missing breakfast causes your body to store additional fat and increases your waistline over time, compared with people who regularly consume a healthy breakfast. As one publication put it, "People who eat breakfast are smarter and skinnier."

Breakfast is also the ideal time to eat protein, which gives you the energy to make it through the day. While sugar-filled cereals and breakfast bars may give you a quick energy boost, the effect does not last. In contrast, eating breakfast foods with a low glycemic index prevents spikes in blood sugar later in the day, which could make for better choices in the afternoon and evening. Instead of traditional cereals for breakfast, consider foods like egg whites, berries, salmon, nuts, seeds, or other options that are not filled with added sugars.

While it's easy to eat well in the morning, it is harder to do as the day progresses. The results of a remarkable study, which aggregated eating habits from 7 million meals worldwide, suggest this problem extends far beyond Western cultures. In every part of the world researchers studied, people's good dietary habits appear to weaken as the sun sets. People make their best food decisions at 7 a.m., get a little worse by 10 a.m., get even worse by 4 p.m., then worsen precipitously by the hour. This occurs because your brain goes into overdrive at the mere sight of high-calorie foods when you are tired. Your brain knows calories will provide energy, which you need more of at 10 p.m., and acts accordingly.

Take a minute to reflect on your own daily eating habits. Eat a healthy breakfast to get your day off to the right start. At lunchtime, opt for greens with a lean form of protein. Avoid meals with fried, fatty, or sugary foods. This will keep your attention and memory sharp throughout the afternoon.

Then rethink the idea of a big traditional dinner. Sitting down with family and friends to have a meal is a great idea. But dinner should not be the meal when you eat substantially larger quantities of food. Your last meal of the day should be the lightest.

Most of us have additional time to plan and prepare a meal in the evening, so try to increase the quality and variety of what you eat for dinner. Use lighter ingredients and smaller portions. Introduce a few new vegetables or spices. Make this the meal where you *learn to enjoy new foods* each day. A lighter dinner will also help you sleep.

Once you have finished your dinner, stop eating. Challenge yourself not to eat *anything* else until breakfast the following day. If you absolutely need a snack before bed, make it small and healthy — perhaps berries, nuts, or apple slices with peanut butter. Then watch out for nights when you stay up much later than usual. As I learned after gaining 40 pounds my first year of college, no good food goes in that late in the day.

◉ ◉ ◉

Television Shortens Your Life Span

It is the path of no resistance; you get home in the evening, sit down, and turn on the television. Before you know it, you have been sitting there watching TV for several hours. While this is the easiest thing to do and watching television is a nice way to unwind, sitting for more than a couple of hours each day can wreak havoc on your health.

Data show that people who spend more than four hours a day watching video are more than twice as likely to have a major cardiac event that kills them or puts them in the hospital, compared with those who spend less than two hours a day on screen-based entertainment. More than four hours of daily television time increases the risk of death from all causes by 48 percent. Even if you are in good general health and exercise regularly, anything beyond two hours of screen time is still bad for your health.

An Australian study of more than 12,000 adults estimated that every single hour spent watching television after the age of 25 decreased the viewer's life expectancy by 22 minutes. For comparison, each cigarette smoked reduces life expectancy by 11 minutes, according to the study's authors. They found that a person who watches six hours of television a day is likely to live about five fewer years than someone who watches no television. Consistent with other findings, these results apply even for people who exercise.

Of course, cutting television out entirely is probably not practical or enjoyable for most people. But if every hour of television is going to cut 22 minutes off your life, at least be selective about what you watch. And when you do watch television, particularly on days when you are less active, get up a few times, add a couple of extra steps, or stretch. Getting up and walking around during commercials could burn an extra 100 calories.

Another option is to save your favorite shows to watch while you exercise. During the winter, I record and then watch a few of my favorite drama series while I'm on my elliptical machine. This gives me even more incentive to drag myself out of bed and work out.

Remember, the main reason researchers study time spent watching television is because it is a good proxy for how much time people spend sitting down. Apparently, it is easier for people to estimate screen time than total sitting time. So if you are watching a movie or show while exercising, it does not count toward the two-hour rule. Be creative and figure out how you can add activity to your TV time.

○ ○ ○

Protect Your Final Hour

For more than a decade, the last thing I did before bed was check my email. I figured it gave me one final chance to make sure everything was taken care of at work before I went to sleep. Unfortunately, this often resulted in my lying in bed thinking about my email exchanges. Particularly when I had been discussing an important topic with someone, the thoughts stuck with me and kept me awake throughout the night.

After realizing how this interfered with my sleep, I imposed a moratorium on checking email right before bed. In reality, there is not much going on after 9 p.m. that can't wait until the next morning. So I gave it a try, and it made a substantive difference right away. It's now been more than a year since I stopped reading email late at night, and my sleep has never been better.

One of the biggest impediments to sleep is what you do in the hour before you go to bed. Checking your messages.

Stressing about your finances. Arguing with a spouse or friend. Watching scary movies. All these things can increase your stress levels at the worst possible time. Then there are other sleep stoppers with direct physical impact, such as drinking too much fluid or eating foods that cause heartburn.

According to a survey from the National Sleep Foundation, roughly two-thirds of people studied do not get enough sleep on weeknights, while more than 90 percent admit using electronic communications in the hour before bed. The light from these devices could suppress your melatonin levels by as much as 20 percent, further disrupting sleep and causing a host of related problems.

To avoid the common sleep saboteurs, establish a ritual so you have at least one hour to unwind before bed each night. Create a mental list of all the things you choose to be off limits during your final hour of the day. Instead of eating, drinking, or using your smartphone, try reading a book or listening to music if it helps you relax.

● ● ●

> Structure your days to eat more early, less late, and nothing after dinner.

> Limit yourself to two hours of *seated* television a day.

> Create a routine so you don't eat, drink, or use electronic messaging in the hour before you go to bed.

Dried and Juiced Is Fruitless

While the pulverized form of a fruit is easy to store and consume on the go, it does not have the same nutritional value as when the fruit is in its whole form. It is easier to give my daughter a juice box than it is to peel a fresh orange. It is more convenient to give my son a box of raisins instead of slicing an apple. However, the *process* of eating and digesting whole foods has great value in itself.

The added fiber from eating a whole fruit and its skin is critical. A single apple has more than *10 times* the fiber of a cup of apple juice. Eating the whole form of fruit also prevents you from overdosing on fructose.

No one sits down to eat 10 apples at one time. However, if you drink a large serving of apple juice, it is easy to consume more sugar than you need in a full day. Most popular juices, such as apple or orange juice, have as much sugar (roughly 10 teaspoons full) as a regular soda. Grape juice contains 15 teaspoons of sugar and is practically liquid candy. A study of more than 250,000 people suggests regular consumption of fruit drinks could be even more detrimental than similar amounts of soda.

When you take these shortcuts and allow a machine's processing to do the work for you, you lose much of the nutritional value of fruit. Dried fruits can be even worse than juice. While the dried form of your favorite fruit may be convenient, you get almost all of the sugar and none of the nutrition.

I have a friend who knows I like to eat healthy, so he used to bring me dried mangoes. Until recently, he did not realize a cup of dried mangoes has 82g of carbohydrates and 76g of sugar. A common candy bar, for comparison, has 26g of carbs and 21g of sugar. The cup of "fruit" has more than *three times* as much sugar as the candy bar.

Dried cranberries and raisins are a common hidden source of sugar in otherwise healthy salads. A single cup of dried cranberries, for example, contains 78g of sugar. When I used the nutritional calculator at one of my favorite lunch spots, I discovered that the raisins took the total sugar content in my salad from 3g to a whopping 30g. One tiny and subtle ingredient ruined the entire meal.

Whenever you have a choice, pick the form of a food closest to the way it was grown originally. The act of eating the whole food will slow your sugar consumption. It will also allow you to get the full nutritional value.

● ● ●

Don't Judge a Box by Its Cover

Potatoes covered in mayonnaise are a type of "salad." Milkshakes are now "smoothies." Sugar water is "vitamin water." Potato chips are rebranded as "veggie chips."

These small marketing tricks are remarkably effective. One study found that dieters are so interested in eating well, they are significantly *more likely* to choose unhealthy foods labeled as healthy. People assume, incorrectly, a dish labeled as a "salad" is somehow healthier than the exact same dish labeled as "pasta." In a similar experiment, participants received samples of a product labeled as either "fruit chews" or "candy chews." Unbeknownst to the participants, they were eating the *exact same food*, just with a different label. Again, dieters perceived the "fruit chews" to be healthier and ate more because of the deceptive labeling.

A few years ago, Kellogg's aired a commercial aimed at selling two of their most sugary cereals, Froot Loops and Apple Jacks, to children. Even though there is no real fruit in these products, that would be nothing new. However, this commercial featured a young boy, dressed up as a doctor, writing a prescription to one of his young friends who apparently needed additional fiber in his diet. The boy dressed up as the doctor proceeded to draw a diagram on the board explaining how the 3 grams of fiber in Froot Loops "makes your tummy happy."

Almost *any* packaged food has some ingredient that *in isolation* is good for your health. Even though the first thing you see on the Froot Loops box is a claim about the 3 grams of added fiber per serving, that claim is not accounting for the 12 grams of sugar or 25 grams of carbohydrates in the same serving. Nor is the box advertising that each serving contains just 1 gram of protein. An egg-white omelet with veggie fillings, for contrast, would have just 3 grams of sugar, only 5 carbs, and 14 grams of protein. In reality, that would make your tummy, brain, and body much happier.

The more claims a product makes, in advertising or packaging, the more you need to be skeptical and ask the right questions. Marketers know that something as simple as using the color green in packaging tricks us into believing that a product has more nutritional value. The foods you should consume are whole fruits and vegetables that will not have extravagant packaging or a national advertising campaign. Cartoon characters on boxes have been shown to mislead parents and children. Deceptive packaging like this helps explain why more than half the foods aimed at children contain excessive sugar.

Make sure to dig at least a few layers beneath the brand name of anything you plan to eat or drink. Don't trust cherry-picked nutritional statistics on the front of the package. It is, after all, in the food producer's best interest to highlight the 3 grams of fiber over the 12 grams of sugar.

◦ ◦ ◦

Make Noise at Night

A few years ago, we purchased our home without realizing the master bedroom was 20 feet away from the back porch of a rental house filled with college students. To counteract the 2 a.m. party music, my wife and I downloaded free white noise apps for our phones to drown out the distraction. It worked remarkably well.

I now use this app whenever I travel. Instead of hearing people in the hallway of my hotel or an elevator closing, all I hear is white noise. Because this is the same sound my brain is used to when I sleep at home, it makes sleeping on the road significantly easier.

Your body essentially tells you to wake up when something unexpected occurs. Whether it is sound, movement, light, or some other form of alarm, most of the things that wake you up at night should not. Loud sounds, from a snoring spouse to a noisy neighbor, are common culprits. They create variance from what your senses expect and ruin your slumber.

Scientists found that the use of constant background noise can be remarkably effective at improving sleep. People who were assigned to sleep in a room with constant noise slept far better when compared with people in a control group who slept in a quiet room. Researchers also noted much higher quality sleep patterns among the people assigned to rooms with constant noise, based on EEG monitoring of brain activity throughout the night.

For those of us with small children, there are periods in life when you *want* to wake up to check if anything is amiss. And if you are camping in a park with grizzly bears, you might not want to use earplugs at night. When you think about these scenarios, you can see why we are alert and vigilant when anything out of the ordinary occurs at night. However, most noises that wake us up today are not critical to our survival.

Eliminate things that could startle you at night. Then escalate the background noise before you go to sleep. Whether you use a noisemaker, a fan, or an app, this noise keeps you from being distracted by subtle disturbances throughout the night. The challenge is to find the right threshold of background volume to keep the unwanted noises out (e.g., an air conditioner kicking in) but not be so loud it keeps you from hearing your smoke alarm or other critical noises.

○ ○ ○

> Replace all dried fruits and fruit juices with whole fruit and other healthy alternatives.

> If you see a packaged food or drink claiming to be healthy on the surface, study all the ingredients in even more detail.

> If sounds wake you up at night, add a constant background noise to keep them from interrupting your sleep. Try a fan, noisemaker, or smartphone app.

Your Routine

Less Heat, Better to Eat

For most of my life, grilling was my method of choice for cooking anything. When I was younger, throwing a burger, steak, or chicken breast on the grill in our backyard was my daily routine. It took little effort to simply turn the gas on, add meat, and wait a few minutes.

Grilling required almost no preparation or cleanup after the fact, compared with other cooking methods. It was quick and simple, and I loved the chargrilled taste of the black crust around the edges. I also assumed grilling was a healthier way to prepare my food. At the time, restaurants were going to great lengths to describe how much healthier grilled options were over fried foods. But it turns out the chargrilled taste is a warning sign for food that is *bad* for your health.

As a new body of research is uncovering, how you *prepare* your food may be as important as the type of food you eat. When you grill, fry, or broil food, the high levels of heat and char produce a class of toxins called advanced glycation end products (AGEs). These AGEs, which are also produced when food is sterilized and pasteurized, have been linked to inflammation, diabetes, obesity, and Alzheimer's, among other health issues.

As a leading medical researcher put it, "Excessive intake of fried, broiled, and grilled foods can overload the body's natural capacity to remove AGEs ... so they accumulate in our tissues, and take over the body's own built-in defenses, pushing them toward a state of inflammation. Over time, this can precipitate disease or early aging."

The challenge is, AGEs are quite deceptive. They often produce desirable smells and tastes. Yet the char that forms when grilling meat in particular is the least healthy part to eat. Anything that creates a crust or crispy border is likely to produce AGEs, which are associated with the type of plaque formation seen in cardiovascular disease. The byproducts wind up on other tissues in the body and cause long-term damage.

While research on the detrimental effects of these cooking methods is in the early stages, other studies make it clear that eating raw or steamed foods helps us retain additional nutrients with each meal. When you have a choice about how your meal is prepared, *prioritize fresh, steamed, or stewed foods ahead of fried, broiled, or grilled.* Avoiding fried foods in particular could have the most rapid return.

Learn to cook with moisture — try steaming, stewing, or poaching — instead of dry heat. Be careful not to over-cook vegetables in particular. If you cook broccoli until it is soft, for example, the health value can plummet. Instead, lightly steam vegetables for a couple of minutes or until they are slightly crunchy. Or simply eat vegetables raw. These basic strategies will help you retain as much of the nutritional value as possible. You may also learn to enjoy the taste of the food you're eating more than the leftover char from a dirty grill.

○ ○ ○

Driving to Divorce

Over the past 50 years, society has had a laser-like focus on determining how we can get from point A to point B as quickly as possible. Perhaps no invention did more to decrease our levels of activity than the automobile. Own-ing a car enables us to build large, less expensive houses in the suburbs. But in turn, we are forced to commute several hours per week. And sitting in a car for all that time is about as sedentary as you can get.

According to one report, the way we have designed our way of life around automobiles could be a leading cause of obesity. After analyzing data collected over a 30-year period, scientists discovered that the correlation between vehicle use and obesity rates was an unusually high 98 percent. While driving is admittedly convenient and the only practical option in many cases, it has a hidden cost.

In one study, when a group of otherwise healthy men were assigned to use crutches and place no weight on one of their legs, it produced swift physiological changes. After just 48 hours, a biopsy of muscle from the inactive leg revealed disruptions in DNA repair, rising oxidative stress, slowing insulin response, and slowing metabolic activity. What's worse, these changes persisted after their activity resumed.

This study suggests that extended periods of inactivity, such as long car rides or flights, could create permanent changes if you get virtually no activity for 24-48 hours. Take small steps, literally, to counteract sedentary days. Get up regularly on long flights. Make stops every couple of hours on road trips. When you arrive at your destination, get some exercise right away. If you have ever spent a few days in a hospital bed, you may have noticed how it takes up to a week or two for your muscles to fully recover from the inactivity.

If you or your spouse is considering a new job opportunity that requires a long commute, give it serious thought. A Swedish study found that couples in which one partner has a commute longer than 45 minutes are a whopping *40 percent more likely to get divorced*. When making a decision about where to live or work, it is easy to underestimate the time you lose with loved ones sitting in a car for an hour or more each day.

A classic study titled *Stress That Doesn't Pay: The Commuting Paradox* found that not even a big pay raise or larger house is worth it if you have to add an hour to your commute. These researchers found that for every extra hour of total commuting time per day, you would need a corresponding 40 percent increase in your salary to make the added car time worthwhile. Whenever you are considering a major move — for school, work, or a new home — start by asking if it will help you spend less time commuting and more time with the people who matter.

If you have no choice but to make an extended daily commute, think about how you could cut back on your total drive time. Could you adjust your work schedule so your commute is during off hours when there is less traffic? Ask your employer if telecommuting is an option one or two days a week. On days when you don't need to physically be in the office — for meetings or other in-person obligations — spending a couple hours in a car is a waste of your time, your well-being, and otherwise productive hours.

◎ ◎ ◎

Sleeping in Only Sounds Good

Breaking the rhythm of your daily routine has consequences. Your body's 24-hour clock, called your circadian rhythm, regulates your sleeping and waking cycles. Each organ has its own circadian clock genes that help you operate with efficiency all day long.

When your biological clock is disrupted (by jet lag, a new shift at work, or eating at a different time), it contributes to a host of issues, from weight gain to heart problems to depression. This may explain why the risk of having a heart attack jumps significantly in the days following time changes due to daylight saving time. Emerging science suggests that disruptions to circadian clock circuitry can even stimulate the onset and progression of cancer. One large-scale study found that people with severe sleep apnea had a 65 percent higher risk of developing cancer. This study alone helped me on a personal level view good sleep as a necessity, not a luxury.

An experiment conducted at Harvard Medical School offers some clues about the way sleep shifting causes serious problems. As part of this carefully controlled study, healthy adults spent five weeks living in a lab. Their sleep patterns were optimal for the first week, then greatly disrupted for three weeks, and intentionally returned to normal in the final recovery phase.

Throughout the disruption phase, participants had just 5.6 hours in bed per 24-hour period. In addition, the timing of participants' sleep schedules was disrupted to simulate real-life events like travel and changing work shifts. As the editor of the medical journal that published this study summarized, "During the 3-week disruption, the participants' glucose control went haywire … this magnitude of disruption … could easily set the stage for development of diabetes and obesity …"

One easy way to keep your clock on track is to wake up at the same time each day. If you can maintain a consistent waking range every day of the week, you are less likely to shift your circadian clock and get out of sync. Maintaining a constant wake-up time will also lead to a stable bedtime. At a minimum, do your best to keep wide time shifts from occurring, even when you travel. While sleeping in on a Sunday always sounds good, the reality is, you pay for it later.

● ● ●

> Steam healthy foods like fish and vegetables instead of grilling them with dry heat.

> Find one way to trim your total weekly transit time, like telecommuting once a week or driving at low-traffic times.

> Wake up at the same general time every day of the week to keep your internal clock on track.

Buy *Use It or Lose It* Foods

In addition to selecting darker colored fruits and vegetables, another quick way to determine if something is good for you is to ask yourself how quickly it spoils. One reason most foods today last longer is because they are chemically modified to spend months in your pantry. Food manufacturers add preservatives because it allows them to extend a product's shelf life. While rice and canned meat may not taste great for eternity, they do have a shelf life of up to five years.

Look at some of the foods that are still hiding on your shelves after months or years. I am guessing you will see rice, pasta, canned goods, bags of flour, sugar, and the like. While some of these are fine to eat on occasion, foods that *do not* last for years on a shelf are usually healthier.

There are always exceptions to this rule of thumb, but to eat right, it takes extra effort to ensure a continuous supply of healthy foods. Go to the grocery store more frequently. Then buy just enough instead of stockpiling as if you were a bear preparing to hibernate for the winter.

After trying this for several years now, I learned that buying more produce frequently also forces me to make better decisions at home. When I see an apple on the counter and know it won't taste as good after a few days, I'm more likely to choose it over a packaged snack. Every time I open our refrigerator and see fresh celery and almond butter, I select that over something like crackers, which will last for several months. Because the healthiest items have immediate "use it or lose it" appeal, I make better daily decisions.

You might need to go shopping every few days instead of stocking up once a month on things you can stow away forever. A little extra effort? Yes. A little extra exercise walking through a grocery store or farmers market more often? Hopefully.

◦ ◦ ◦

How You Move Matters

A young woman is so engrossed in texting, she falls into a shallow pool of water in the middle of a shopping mall. A man walks directly into a post while reading his email on a smartphone. Perhaps you have seen one of these online videos. Incidents like this will only become more common. They can even put you in danger when pedestrians and drivers fail to pay attention to their surroundings.

As you walk by people on the street or in the hallway, study the way they carry themselves. Observe their posture. Notice how often people keep their head down and slump as they walk. Or you might notice how fixated people are with handheld devices as they risk pedestrian collisions to read their messages.

This "smartphone pose" is bad for your wrists, neck, and back. I forced myself to stop using my smartphone while walking a few years ago. It not only reduced my back pain but also allowed me to focus on my natural surroundings and take a break from the reactionary world of email.

The next time you're walking in a public area, keep your gadgets in your pocket, your back straight, and your chin and head above your shoulders looking forward. Practice walking tall. Notice how much better it feels for your back and body when your head is not facing down with your arm and wrist curled.

Beyond the obvious physical problems, poor posture also makes a bad impression on others. People who are simply asked to adopt dominant poses feel more in control and do a better job of handling stress, according to one study. Adopting a powerful pose also minimizes physical pain.

The next time you want to project confidence, stand, walk, or sit up straight. To maintain better posture, remind yourself to keep your ears directly above your shoulders and your shoulders directly above your hips as much as possible. Maintaining this alignment can improve muscle tone, decrease pain, and even make it easier to breathe.

◉ ◉ ◉

Keep Stress From Ruining Your Sleep

Stress leads to a lot of lost sleep over time. But it's hard to shut off those stressors that keep you up at night right before bed. What you can do is get ahead of stressors before they occur. When researchers study people who are successful at minimizing their stress levels, they find things like breathing exercises help a little. Yet of all the stress management techniques I studied, one in particular is the most effective: prevention.

Stress prevention starts with structuring your days to *avoid situations likely to cause stress before they occur*. This is far more effective than deep breathing or counting to 10 in the midst of a stressful situation. I don't mean you should skip getting married, working, or having kids to avoid stress. The best way to avoid stress is to prevent smaller daily stressors in advance.

It is critical you get ahead of this cycle because poor sleep puts additional stress on your immune system. This stress makes you more likely to get common ailments like a cold or the flu. Scientists are learning more about this topic, and chronic stress may even have dire consequences, such as fueling the metastasis of certain cancers.

After learning just how damaging stress and sleeplessness are on the body, I made a series of changes to my own routine. This knowledge motivated me to structure my days for less stress. When I traveled, I left earlier for the airport so I was not worried about missing my flight. When a discussion got heated at work, I took a step back to put things in perspective.

Last year, I realized the biggest stressor in my life was that I could not find time to work on a project I was deeply passionate about: this book. The stress from *not* doing something I care about this deeply was keeping me up most nights. So I made a major career change and left a job I loved to spend all my time working on this book. Almost immediately after making this decision, the stress and sleepless nights ended.

Identify what stressors are keeping you up at night, big or small. Tackle the big ones first. Then find the smaller irritants and fix them. If you can plan your days to minimize recurrent stressors, you will have much better nights of sleep.

An interesting finding from recent research is that the way you *deal with stress* can be more important than the stressor itself. If you get overly upset by daily stressors and continue to dwell on them after the fact, your health will suffer. However, if you make the decision to accept what happened and let it go quickly, it reduces the long-term damage to your health and well-being. In reality, most daily stressors will not matter much a year from now, which is always a helpful reminder. So the next time something causes you undue stress, remember that *your reaction matters more than the stressful event itself.*

○ ○ ○

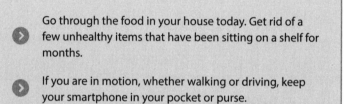

Go through the food in your house today. Get rid of a few unhealthy items that have been sitting on a shelf for months.

If you are in motion, whether walking or driving, keep your smartphone in your pocket or purse.

Identify one thing that stresses you out regularly. Create a plan to prevent it from occurring in the first place.

Get a Tan From Tomatoes

Whether you realize it or not, you make quick assumptions about how healthy someone is based on his or her physical appearance. Or you may have noticed how easy it is to spot a person who smokes by his extensive wrinkles and skin damage. In direct contrast, you can see the increased blood flow and vibrancy in the faces of your friends who eat well and work out each morning. As it turns out, you are what you eat, and *you look like what you eat*.

In a novel experiment, a team of researchers in Europe found that people who ate additional portions of fruits and vegetables were rated by others as having a healthier glow. People with this "dietary tan" were even rated by third-party observers as looking healthier than people who got a tan from natural sunlight. As Dr. Ian Stephen put it, "Most people think the best way to improve skin color is to get a suntan, but our research shows that eating lots of fruits and vegetables is actually more effective." The researchers attributed this increased vibrancy in skin tone to the effect of carotenoids, which are abundant in vegetables like tomatoes and carrots in particular.

What you eat also affects the quality of your hair (or lack thereof). Hair grows on average about half an inch every month, and the nutrients you eat serve as the foundation for all new hair, skin, and nail growth. Foods likely to increase the health and thickness of hair include blueberries, salmon, spinach, and walnuts. The key is to have an overall balanced diet with the right nutrients.

● ● ●

Look Younger With Each Step

Physical activity does as much for your exterior as it does for your interior. Researchers study the physical impact of various conditions in the lab using mice. They use mice to determine how certain drugs or activities could affect humans, for better or worse. Even though these studies sometimes fail to translate in human trials, a recent experiment on activity and aging offers tantalizing clues for all of us.

In this experiment, a team of researchers genetically programmed a group of mice to grow old at a much more rapid pace than normal. The mice that did *not* exercise over the first eight months (the equivalent age of early 60s in human years) became extremely frail and decrepit. They had smaller muscles and brains, enlarged hearts, shrunken gonads, and hair that turned patchy and gray. This group of mice could barely move around their cages, and *all of them died* before reaching one year of age.

Another group of mice genetically programmed to age rapidly were allowed to run on a wheel for 45 minutes three times a week, starting at three months of age (the equivalent of age 20 in human years). The mice continued with this vigorous exercise (human equivalent of 18 miles per week) for the next five months. By the eight month mark, unlike their sedentary peers, the mice that exercised maintained full pelts of dark fur (no graying), kept their muscle mass and brain volume, and had normal gonads and hearts. At one year, *none of the mice that exercised had died* from natural causes. As lead researcher Dr. Mark Tarnopolsky summarized, "Exercise alters the course of aging."

It is important to note these 45-minute exercise sessions were at a fairly strenuous pace. The human equivalent would be running about 6 miles at an 8-9 minute-per-mile pace three days a week. If you are in good shape and prefer to get your vigorous exercise in a few intensive sessions per week, this might be a good option. But even Dr. Tarnopolsky was unsure this pace would be necessary for humans to see benefits. He suggests that people who have been inactive should start with five minutes of walking per day, then gradually increase their activity level.

Increased exercise has produced similar results in human trials and works at any age. Even among heart failure patients over 65, regular aerobic activity counteracts muscle breakdown, increases strength, and decreases inflammation caused by aging. No matter what your age or current physical condition is, moving more will keep you looking and feeling younger.

◉ ◉ ◉

Sleep to Impress

The vibrancy of a person's face shapes our immediate perception. I will admit, as I meet and interact with people, my mind is constantly making snap judgments. If a colleague's face looks wiped out and he has dark circles under his eyes, I make assumptions, even if they are incorrect or unfair. My first reaction is usually empathetic because I can relate to sleepless nights.

However, my mind sometimes makes less forgiving interpretations as well. When I spot a sleep-deprived colleague, I wonder if he has enough energy to make a meaningful contribution to a meeting. What's worse, if I notice a pattern, I assume he is struggling more generally at work or in his personal life. Others may suspect a drinking problem. Again, none of this is particularly fair, but we make these snap judgments hundreds of times in a week.

Nothing is more damaging to the way others perceive us as the cosmetic impact of sleep deprivation. A study published in the *British Medical Journal* found that random people clearly judge us based on how sleepy or rested we look. What the researchers learned, after asking 65 untrained observers to rate photos of people who were sleep deprived versus those with normal sleep, confirms what you would have guessed.

Without any background knowledge, random people rated the "sleep-deprived" group as being less healthy, less attractive, and more tired. Other studies reveal that the stress-induced changes associated with insomnia could cause your skin to look much worse through various physiological mechanisms.

Sleeplessness is one of the only major conditions visible on the outside *before* it takes a long-term toll inside.

On days when you need the most energy and want to make a good physical impression, plan for a sound night of sleep. If you sleep well consistently over time, it will cut years off your appearance.

○ ○ ○

> Eat more carrots and tomatoes for a truly natural tan. Also add salmon and blueberries for better hair and skin.

> Walk at least five minutes a day to counteract aging. Build up to 45 minutes of intense activity at least three days a week to halt aging even more.

> When you need to look your best, give yourself plenty of time to get a sound night's sleep.

An Extra Boost

Eat the Healthiest Food First

My four-year-old daughter loves pasta, which is not the healthiest food. I noticed she was eating and filling up on the pasta first then leaving most of the vegetables on her plate. So instead of being a militant parent and taking away pasta altogether, I told her she could have it *after* she finished her vegetables. While she might not enjoy broccoli as much as macaroni, she now finishes her vegetables every time and leaves some pasta behind.

My wife and I tried following the same rule and found it worked for us as well. When I go out to dinner, most meals start with a big salad. When my entrée arrives, I start with the vegetables. Eating the healthiest foods first also makes it easier to resist the temptation of dessert.

As research over the last decade has revealed, the dish you start with serves as an anchor food for your entire meal. Experiments show that people eat nearly 50 percent greater quantity of the food they eat first. If you start with a dinner roll, you will eat more starches, less protein, and fewer vegetables. Beginning your meal with a starch also makes you likely to eat more overall.

Eat the healthiest food on your plate first. As age-old wisdom suggests, this usually means starting with your vegetables or salad. If you are going to eat something unhealthy, at least save it for last. This will give your body the opportunity to fill up on better options before you move on to starches, carbs, or sugary desserts. It will also ensure you eat larger quantities of what is best for you.

When you expect to be tempted with bad choices, try *priming before a meal* with healthy alternatives. Find something healthy to fill your stomach a little and decrease your appetite. One study revealed simply drinking a large glass of water before each meal resulted in significant weight loss over time.

A strategy that worked for me is eating a small snack before going somewhere where healthy options could be limited. If I am going to a friend's house who usually serves meat and pasta, I load up on nuts or veggies before

I leave home. This makes it much easier to avoid overindulging later.

○ ○ ○

The Right Way to Get High

Think about the most enjoyable forms of exercise you have ever experienced. This could be any activity — for example, running, biking, football, soccer, tennis, yoga, or Pilates. Within that specific type of workout, see if you can identify some of the best moments in particular.

For me, there is a point around two miles into an outdoor run at which the activity is far more enjoyable. Any aches and pains from the first minutes of running are gone. My heart rate and breathing are at a sustainable level. The endorphins are kicking in and giving me a natural high.

When scientists study this phenomenon, they find that this pleasurable moment usually occurs at or before you reach your "ventilatory threshold," which is *the point when breathing is so difficult it is hard to talk*. While a few people feel their best after this threshold, for most of us, it is near or just before this point.

You have an evolutionary addiction to exercise. Our early ancestors had to chase their next meal on foot and run away from predators. Scientists speculate that this is why the so-called "runner's high" became part of our evolution.

Researchers are uncovering how and when this natural high occurs. Intense activity triggers the release of brain chemicals called endocannabinoids, which create a potent feeling of pleasure. When this is tested in the lab by having people either walk or run on a treadmill for 30 minutes, running more than doubles the level of endocannabinoids released in the brain. As one physician described what occurs when she runs, "When you first start, you feel a little stiff ... but then once you get started, everything loosens up ... Your heart gets stronger. It gets bigger. The amount of blood your heart can pump is more."

Walking is beneficial to your health, but it does not provide the same high as running does. Jogging a few times a week can also add five to six years to your life, but that is not a great motivator to go for a run tomorrow. If you want an immediate high, get 30 minutes of high-intensity exercise.

● ● ●

Sleep Your Way to a New Day

If you have a lousy day, deep REM (rapid eye movement) sleep may be your best defense so the next day is better. A team of Berkeley researchers discovered that during REM sleep, your stress chemistry shuts down so your brain can process emotional experiences. This deep sleep takes the edge off difficult memories. As one of the researchers stated, "During REM sleep, memories are being reactivated, put in perspective and connected and integrated, but in a state where stress neurochemicals are beneficially suppressed."

To test this, the scientists divided people into two groups who viewed 150 emotional images 12 hours apart while a functional MRI (fMRI) scanner measured their brain activity. Half of the participants viewed the images in the morning and then again in the evening (meaning they stayed awake between the two viewings). The other half viewed the images for the first time in the evening then again the next morning (so this group slept for much of the 12-hour period between viewings instead of staying awake).

Members of the group who slept between image viewings reported a significant decrease in their emotional reaction to the images. The fMRI scans of this group also revealed a dramatic reduction in reactivity in the brain's amygdala, the region that processes emotions. The group who slept between scans also had significant decreases in levels of stress neurochemicals in the brain.

As this experiment illustrates, your deepest period of sleep serves as "REM therapy" for processing traumatic events without producing damaging stress neurochemicals and hormones. At the end of a difficult day, remind yourself how a good night of sleep can accelerate your recovery. Think of sleeping like being anesthetized for surgery. It allows your brain to do the difficult work with less pain.

When you manage to get a decent night of sleep, you can start the next day with less burden from the prior day's events. Even if you are not "back to normal" the next morning, you're likely in a much better place than before you went to bed. At best, it feels like a new day.

○ ○ ○

> Start every meal with the *most* healthy item on your plate, and end with the *least*.

> Identify one aerobic activity that gives you a natural high. Do it at least once a week for 30 minutes.

> At the end of a lousy day, before you make a small stressor into something bigger, give sleep a chance to do some repair work overnight.

Grab a Handful

Think about the last time you ate at your desk while working, had a meal while watching television, or dined while driving. I'm guessing you ate more than you planned and enjoyed your meal less. A Harvard study found that people consumed 167 *additional* calories per hour while watching television.

I have a real weakness for dark chocolate almonds. In the past, I would grab the entire container, take it with me, and sit in front of the television. Even though I told myself I would only eat a few, that inevitably turned into 20 before I put the container away. Recently, I decided to discipline myself on this occasional indulgence. I now force myself to grab a portion no larger than a single handful and leave the container in the pantry. This simple change cut my consumption by two-thirds.

Instead of multitasking while eating, focus on what and how much goes in your mouth with each bite. Avoid checking messages, reading, or watching a show while you eat. If you can't help but snack while multitasking, trick yourself into slowing down.

When a team of researchers studied consumption habits of people eating popcorn in a movie theater, they discovered that good or poor taste had little bearing on how much popcorn participants consumed. Even though no one likes week-old popcorn, the participants who were used to eating popcorn in a movie theater consumed just as much whether it was fresh or stale. But the most interesting part of this experiment was what happened when researchers instructed these moviegoers to eat with only their non-dominant hand. Using the less familiar hand, study participants ate considerably less popcorn.

Another study suggests even subtle "stop signs" can curb a binge. When researchers placed one red potato chip for every 5 or 10 regular colored chips in a stack, it reduced consumption significantly. On average, participants ate about 50 percent less when these subconscious stop signs were in place, even though they were not told the red chip's hidden purpose.

Apparently, we just need something to help us remember to pause. To get ahead of unintentional binge eating, limit yourself to one handful when you reach for a snack. Or put a predetermined portion on a plate, napkin, or bowl. This will allow *you to set the amount* you plan to consume in advance. Then you don't need to worry about getting so engrossed in what you're doing that you forget to stop eating. Another option is to snack on something that requires work to eat, like pistachios in the shell. When you have to work for it or think about it, you eat less.

○ ○ ○

Take Five Outside

Outdoor activity gives you a little extra kick. A series of studies revealed that exercising in a natural environment yields more benefit than indoor workouts. Outdoor activity leads to increased energy, positive emotions, and feelings of revitalization. It can even decrease tension, confusion, anger, and depression.

Participants in these studies reported greater enjoyment and satisfaction with outdoor activity. They were also more likely to repeat the activity. Even if you need to bundle up at certain times of the year, it is worth battling the cold.

I often feel the need to get out of my house or office after a full day indoors. Even when I've had ample indoor exercise, there's something about a natural environment that boosts my energy. An hour on the treadmill pales in comparison to an hour of walking around my neighborhood.

The good news is, just *five minutes of outdoor activity* is all you need to boost your mood. The study that produced this discovery also concluded that any outdoor activity — walking, gardening, cycling, or fishing — will do the trick. Better yet, merge a few minutes outdoors with social time. If you have kids, go out and play ball. Take a brief walk with a colleague to grab a coffee. Go on a neighborhood walk with your significant other in the morning or evening. Walk your dog. Remember, even quick outings are beneficial on cold days.

Any environment should work, from a nature trail to an urban street. On days when you are in danger of getting almost no outdoor time, step out for a brief walk. It will yield real benefits for your mental and physical health.

● ● ●

Pay for Peer Pressure

Having another person hold you accountable is a great way to get and stay in shape. As busy as people are today, we often need a little "nudge," as behavioral economists call it, to be more active. This accountability is one of the primary reasons people spend money on personal trainers or commit to group classes and activities. They know that someone else will be counting on them to show up and they have already made the financial investment.

A new series of studies found that the effect of even occasional nudges has a lasting impact. Researchers at Stanford recruited 218 people and divided them into three groups. All participants were told they should have a goal of walking half an hour on most days. The first group served as a control, the second group received automated messages every three weeks asking about their exercise patterns, and the third group received calls from a person who stayed in touch and encouraged them throughout the year-long study. Those who received the calls from a live person were congratulated on any exercise they performed and encouraged to do more in the future.

After 12 months, all three groups showed some improvement, perhaps because they knew there would be follow-up at the end of the study. The group who received no regular phone calls reported exercising for about two hours per week at the end of the year-long study. People who received automated calls and encouragement exercised just over two and a half hours per week. The group who spoke to a live person every three weeks went from just over an hour and a half of weekly exercise at the start of the study to almost three hours per week by the time the study wrapped up.

A simple check-in from another person nearly doubled each participant's activity over the span of a year. As one of the Stanford researchers explained, it often takes more than individual willpower to change behavior, "Whether it's smoking or alcohol use or physical inactivity, social support helps prevent against relapse ... a light touch can have lasting effect." This study and many others suggest that almost anyone, even someone you don't know well, can help hold you accountable.

That being said, having a close friend nudge you in the right direction can be even more helpful. If you plan to exercise with a friend for motivation, research suggests you will benefit more if your friend is better than you at a given activity. Peers who perform better yet give you less verbal encouraging during the workout (presumably to avoid being condescending) are more effective.

If you don't have someone who encourages you to be healthier today, find at least one person to help you reach a specific health goal. This person doesn't need to check in on you every day. It could be a friend, colleague, sibling, spouse, or anyone else who is willing to help. If you're more comfortable hiring a personal trainer or using an online system, this can work and be well worth the investment. Just make sure you have a mechanism in place to have someone remind you of your health goals and check in on how you are doing every once in a while.

○ ○ ○

> When you want a quick snack, take a handful and leave the bag or box behind.

> Spend at least five minutes outside every day.

> Identify one person who will check in regularly and hold you accountable for staying active. This could be a friend, coach, or personal trainer.

Prevention

25

Eat to Beat Cancer

Half of all men and one-third of all women in America will be diagnosed with cancer. Even if you are not formally diagnosed, you probably have microscopic cancer cells in your body that are too small to see on an MRI or CT scan. When researchers conduct autopsies of people who die in car accidents, for example, they often find undiagnosed cancers. According to one leading researcher, microscopic cancers are likely forming in our bodies all the time.

Most of these microscopic cancers never grow large enough to pose a threat. They sit dormant in the organ where they live, as small as the tip of a ballpoint pen, lacking an adequate blood supply. This is where your lifestyle and diet play a major role, for better or worse.

What you eat can greatly reduce the risk of cancers growing and spreading. Diet and physical activity have been shown to reduce recurrences of cancer and to extend survival. In my own experience, many of my largest tumors have not changed in size over the last decade. While there is no way to know how much my dietary changes have slowed this growth over time, they certainly help my odds.

Maintaining a lean body weight is a good place to start to curb cancerous growth. According to recent studies, obesity acts as a "bona fide tumor promoter." Obesity creates a chronic inflammatory state that makes it easier for cancer to grow and spread throughout the body.

Epidemiological studies suggest that obese people have about a 50 percent increase in their risk for all cancers. For specific types of cancer, such as liver cancer, the risk for people who are obese goes up by as much as 450 percent. It appears maintaining a normal weight may be one of the best things you can do to minimize your long-term risk of cancer.

To prevent the growth and spread of cancerous cells in your body, consume more of these foods and drinks: apples, artichokes, blueberries, bok choy, broccoli, green tea, kale, lemons, mushrooms, raspberries, red grapes, red wine, salmon, strawberries, and tomatoes. Also consider eating ingredients commonly used for flavor that have cancer-fighting potential: cinnamon, garlic, nutmeg, parsley, and turmeric.

Try these foods and spices as replacements for sweet or fried foods. Also watch out for processed meats, red meat, saturated fats, and added sugar. All of these food types have been linked to increased cancer rates in different parts of the body. While no diet alone will prevent or cure cancer, you can absolutely *decrease the odds* of cancer by eating the right foods. If you feed your body well, you may starve cancer in the process.

○ ○ ○

Get a Prescription for Exercise

Taking a pill should be your last resort, not your first line of defense. We are often quick to jump to one of the many answers that arrive in the form of a pill. While medications are often essential and reduce the near-term risk of life-threatening events, they are not always the right long-term solution.

In the words of medical researcher Alex Clark, who studies the effect of exercise on heart function, *"Exercise is a wonder drug that hasn't been bottled."* Exercise could be as effective as medication for treating everything from depression to migraines. Friends of mine who have battled depression swear regular activity is one of their best defenses. Added activity can also help you use fewer over-the-counter pain medications by decreasing inflammation.

I know from my own experience that exercising is the best way to keep chronic pain at bay. Activity does more to reduce my back and neck pain than any drug I have tried. I have also found vigorous exercise to be far more effective than pharmaceutical remedies for improving the quality of my sleep. As a result of increasing my activity in recent years, I was able to eliminate almost all prescription and over-the-counter drugs.

Regular activity also modifies your genes in a way that could benefit your diet. When scientists analyzed people's DNA before and after half an hour of exercise, they found that the activity altered the way DNA produces specialized muscle proteins that boost metabolism. This change caused the muscles to burn more fats and sugars, which could reduce the need for a variety of medications that help the body compensate for poor dietary choices.

The next time you visit your doctor, ask about some of the medications you could reduce or even eliminate if you had enough activity in your daily regimen. Or just boost your activity levels, and see if it starts to alleviate your symptoms. It may turn out you need a prescription for exercise more than you need the latest pharmacological solution.

Know Two Numbers by Heart

Despite the fact heart disease kills millions worldwide every year, it is one of the most preventable ailments ever studied. A landmark international study dubbed Interheart compared people on every continent who suffered a heart attack with a similar number of relatives who did not. After studying more than 15,000 people across continents, this study determined that about *90 percent of the risk associated with a heart attack is within your control.*

High cholesterol, blood pressure, physical activity, smoking, and diet all have a profound influence on the likelihood of developing heart disease. The most important thing is to prevent a heart attack before it occurs. Once you've had a heart attack, the odds of dying in the next year soar. In the year following a recognized heart attack, 25 percent of men and 38 percent of women will die. This is why you need to get ahead of your heart health before it is too late.

Start by knowing two fundamental metrics: your cholesterol and your blood pressure. As one article put it, knowing these numbers "is as fundamental to heart health as knowing the alphabet is to reading." With cholesterol, look at the balance of good (HDL) versus bad (LDL) metrics in particular, as total cholesterol can be misleading. Unfortunately, many people don't even know their own numbers, let alone how those numbers compare to what is ideal. At a minimum, track these numbers annually — and more frequently if you have any type of elevated risk for heart disease.

While getting your cholesterol checked usually requires a blood test and a doctor visit, checking your blood pressure is much easier. It is also less expensive. Home blood pressure monitors start at about $20. If you are into higher-tech solutions, there are blood pressure cuffs that connect to your smartphone for regular tracking. A more cost-effective solution is to visit your local drug store, pharmacy, or even grocery store. They often have a professional-grade station where you can check your blood pressure for free.

If you eat well and don't smoke, it is much less likely you will need to use drugs to manage your blood pressure or cholesterol. Start by improving your diet to keep these numbers in check. Then try to get 30 minutes of exercise each day, which is associated with a 70 percent reduction in the risk of a heart attack. If 30 minutes is not possible on some days, at least take a 10-minute walk.

When scientists at the Mayo Clinic analyzed data on this topic, they found that even a brisk 10-minute walk each day results in a nearly 50 percent reduction in heart attack risk, compared with people who get hardly any exercise. A little activity can even help raise your good cholesterol. Also watch out for simply sitting too much. According to the Mayo Clinic study, sitting is about the same as smoking when it comes to increasing your risk for heart disease.

○ ○ ○

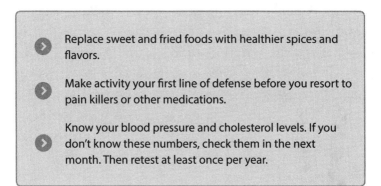

> Replace sweet and fried foods with healthier spices and flavors.

> Make activity your first line of defense before you resort to pain killers or other medications.

> Know your blood pressure and cholesterol levels. If you don't know these numbers, check them in the next month. Then retest at least once per year.

Daily Choices

Buy Willpower at the Store

The most influential choices you make for your health occur in the grocery store. Once you put something in your cart, good or bad, it is likely to end up in your stomach. Even if you feel some remorse about your poor choice in the store, when you get home, your willpower stands little chance. After all, you paid for it, and it is only a few steps away at that point.

One of my vices is Wheat Thins crackers. If I can find them at home, I will eat the entire box, usually in a day or two. Because these crackers are loaded with carbohydrates and salt, they have an addictive taste that makes it almost impossible for me to eat just one or two. My limited willpower is no match. I finally realized the only way to win this battle is to make sure the box of Wheat Thins never makes its way into my house.

To get ahead of my temptation to purchase snack crackers at the grocery store, I use Amazon's "subscribe and save" feature for healthier items. Every month, they send me a fresh supply of nuts, green tea, and other healthy snacks. Allowing this subscription to renew also makes these choices more automatic.

Anytime I visit our neighborhood grocery store, I spend most of my time in the fresh produce and seafood sections. I also try to avoid the middle aisles altogether, as they are filled with unhealthy and addictive items. If I don't see the salty pretzels (another major vice), there is no chance they will wind up in my cart.

Being aware of your own temptations gives you an opportunity to get ahead. When you are at the store, put the right things in your cart so bad choices don't make the trip home. Better yet, make a list of healthy foods to buy in *advance* so you are less likely to load up on poor impulse choices.

When it is practical, shop for food when you are full. As your hunger increases, the quality of your dietary decisions decreases. If you walk through the aisles of the store hungry, you will fill your cart with less healthy foods. Get in the habit of shopping for food after, not before, your normal mealtime. If you get ahead of your own hunger instinct, you will make better purchasing decisions. Then at home, it will take less willpower to eat well every day.

Clean Your Brain and Bowels

Some of the greatest benefits of exercise are hiding beneath the surface. As scientists learn more, it appears exercise can "speed the removal of garbage from inside our body's cells." Studies suggest that regular exercise helps the cells inside your body sweep away debris, such as viruses and bacteria, that accumulate over time.

Daily workouts may even help clear debris from your brain. A series of laboratory experiments with animals found that regular exercise *reverses* the adverse effects of a high-fat diet on the brain. These studies suggest that exercise stimulates the production of substances in the brain that degrade the plaques associated with Alzheimer's disease.

Fortunately, the amount of exercise that protected the brains of lab rats and mice is equivalent to about a 30-minute run for humans. Any vigorous activity should do the trick. You don't need to be a long-distance runner to get these benefits from exercise. As long as your body is literally in motion for a few hours a day, it keeps things from slowing down, clogging up, and settling in.

Researchers are only scratching the surface in terms of the mechanisms through which exercise benefits your well-being. However, it is clear that activity not only gives you extra energy, but it also clears out your system. This helps explain why experts recommend regular exercise to avoid constipation and to maintain regularity.

If you have ever tried running a longer distance than normal, you might have noticed how the up-and-down motion of running rattles things loose inside. There is a reason why marathon routes are lined with portable restrooms. Between this and the sweat you produce during intense activity, exercising is one of the most rapid ways to keep your body from clogging up and slowing down.

○ ○ ○

Sleep on It

When you need to make a big decision, do it after a sound night of sleep. One experiment showed just how important sleep is if you want to learn and make good decisions. When people in this study learned a new technique for winning a game *in the evening* then went home to sleep on it, they made much better decisions in the morning when they returned.

In comparison, people in the study who did the same activity *in the morning* and had a waking day to think on it did poorly. The group who *slept* made better decisions *four times* as often compared with the group who had all those waking hours to think on it.

Fortunately, when people are asked to solve easier problems, a full night of sleep makes no difference. As a researcher who has studied this topic said, "Our study shows that this sleep effect is greatest when the problems facing us are difficult. Sleep appears to help us solve problems by accessing information that is remote to the initial problem, that may not be initially brought to mind."

The age-old axiom "Sleep on it" is based in good science. The next time you need to solve a difficult problem or have a major life decision to make, give it the time and sleep it deserves.

○ ○ ○

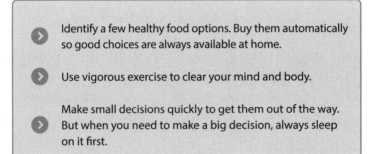

Identify a few healthy food options. Buy them automatically so good choices are always available at home.

Use vigorous exercise to clear your mind and body.

Make small decisions quickly to get them out of the way. But when you need to make a big decision, always sleep on it first.

Save the Cake for *Your* Birthday

Every day is someone's birthday. If you have ever worked in an office, you likely noticed there are several "special occasions" in any given week warranting candy, pastries, or cake. While celebrating birthdays, anniversaries, holidays, and other milestones is healthy, using them as an excuse for eating sugar and refined carbs is not. What's worse, our flawed mental accounting allows us to conveniently forget these "exceptions," even though we might have consumed enough sugar for the entire day.

Eventually, workplaces and gathering spots will have better options for these types of celebrations. Until social expectations start to change, define what is truly a special occasion. There are always reasons to indulge, and it's fine to do so occasionally, but save it for your own birthday instead of every coworker's.

The environment you create in your home could be even more important than broader cultural influences. One of the most effective ways to help obese adults and children lose weight is through a process researchers call "family-based behavioral treatment." The key to this treatment working *for the child* is that *the parent loses weight*. A parent's weight loss is the only factor that predicts the child's weight loss.

Figure out what you can do to improve unhealthy family rituals. Eating as a family at home, instead of dining out, is a good start. If meals in your home revolve around fried foods, refined carbohydrates, or other unhealthy foods, slowly turn the tide. Think about eliminating sweets if dessert is a ritual every night. For those of you with children, consider the message it sends when you *reward* kids with ice cream if they eat their veggies. At a minimum, add some healthy options so your family has a chance to make better choices.

Substitute a bowl of fresh fruit or berries for dessert. Mix in some unsweetened coconut or flax milk, and you have a relatively healthy alternative with a naturally sweet taste. Research has shown that a variety of berries, blueberries and strawberries in particular, serve as a "natural housekeeper" for your health. Berries have diverse antioxidant mechanisms linked to better brain health, lower risk of diabetes, and decreased risk of Parkinson's disease. One report describes how berry fruits actually change the way neurons in your brain communicate. These changes in signaling can prevent inflammation in the brain and improve motor control and thinking.

Most restaurants that serve dessert also have fruit or berries on hand. They are usually not on the menu as standalone items, but that should not prevent you from ordering them when you dine out. My late grandfather used to ask for a bowl of berries as his dessert whenever we went to a restaurant. Every time I watched him try this, the restaurant figured out a way to make it work, and he got berries or fruit *without* the ice cream.

Raspberries, blackberries, and acai berries are other healthy options for a creative dessert. One challenge is finding berries during off seasons. If fresh berries are not available, try the frozen variety. Another option is to make desserts from common fruits you can find year-round, like apples and bananas. Remember, almost any natural choice is better than cake or ice cream.

○ ○ ○

Indulge Less to Enjoy More

When you indulge, you enjoy the fifteenth bite far less than the first. A rare treat increases your happiness more than daily indulgence in that same treat. There is something about maintaining novelty that could improve your health and well-being at the same time.

As part of an experiment, one group of chocolate lovers was assigned to eat a piece of chocolate, then they pledged *not to eat any more* for the next week. A second group of chocolate lovers ate the initial chocolate then were told *to eat as much as they wanted* over the span of a week. The second group was even given a two-pound bag of chocolate to help them achieve this "goal."

When both groups returned a week later, the participants who continued to consume chocolate on a daily basis enjoyed it significantly less. In contrast, the participants who ate no chocolate during the week enjoyed it as much as ever. *Giving up* a favorite indulgence for a week helped chocolate lovers *renew their enjoyment*.

If you can't imagine life without chocolate, the good news is, eating a little dark chocolate has some health benefits. Small portions of dark chocolate could reduce the risk of heart attack and stroke. Milk chocolate, the most common type, did not have the same effect, and white chocolate had no benefit at all. Even dark chocolate is a bad idea if it has any type of sugar-based filling.

Limit yourself to one or two small squares of dark chocolate to keep the good effects from outweighing the bad. Challenge yourself to let one bar of chocolate last a few weeks. At least try not to eat an entire bar in one sitting. If you are like me and need help to overcome a lack of willpower, buy individually wrapped chocolate squares to keep yourself from conveniently losing count. Look for dark chocolate with at least 70 percent cocoa and little added sugar, as these varieties contain additional flavonoids and have greater cardiovascular benefits.

The same indulgence effect is likely to hold true for other foods and drinks. If you drink your favorite wine every week, it is sure to be less enjoyable than if you save it for special occasions. When you plan to indulge in a food or drink, find a way to ration the amount and frequency of what you consume. Order the smallest possible serving of ice cream. Or share one of your favorite treats with someone else so you both get a few bites. If you keep servings small and indulgences rare, you will have less guilt, more enjoyment, and better health.

○ ○ ○

Take Credit to Make It Count

Tracking all of your activity, in itself, improves objective physical health outcomes. While just *knowing* how much activity you get would not seem likely to change your *actual* health, it might. A fascinating study conducted by a team of Harvard researchers explored the impact of *simply telling* a group of housekeepers how many calories they burn during the day.

To study this objectively, the researchers divided hotel housekeepers into two groups. They told the first group that the work they do each day, cleaning hotel rooms, is good exercise and satisfies the surgeon general's recommendations for an active lifestyle. They also gave this group examples of how their daily work *was* exercise. The researchers followed the other group of housekeepers for the same period of time. These housekeepers performed the same daily activities as the first group. But they were *not given any information about the value of their exercise.*

Four weeks later, the housekeepers who received information about the value of their daily activity weighed less and had lower blood pressure, lower body fat, a smaller waist-to-hip ratio, and a lower body mass index. The control group did not see any such gains, even though they continued the same activity throughout the four-week study. It was clear the additional information researchers provided to the first group created a sort of placebo effect that improved *real and objective health outcomes.*

Think through your daily activities and identify exercise that your mental accounting is missing. Then as you do basic tasks like yard work or cleaning the house, keep in mind the value they add for your overall health. Better yet, use a pedometer to see exactly how much you are moving throughout the day. When you can see these little things adding up, it improves your actual health. The more credit you take, the more benefit you get.

Next, add a few "microactivities" to your routine. Think of microactivities as *any movements that make a measurable contribution to your health but would not count as a full workout.* These seemingly small activities have been shown to add up and benefit our health in the long term. Consider all the opportunities you have, for example: a little time cleaning the house, making an extra trip up the stairs, or walking to the printer at work. Even subtle activities matter.

○ ○ ○

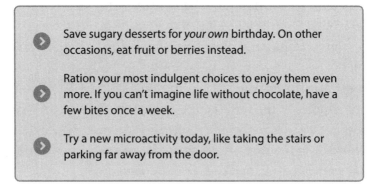

> Save sugary desserts for *your own* birthday. On other occasions, eat fruit or berries instead.

> Ration your most indulgent choices to enjoy them even more. If you can't imagine life without chocolate, have a few bites once a week.

> Try a new microactivity today, like taking the stairs or parking far away from the door.

Broccoli Is the New Black

You know broccoli is good for you. Maybe you even eat it a few times a week, despite the inclinations of your taste buds. I was never a big fan of broccoli myself, but as I read more about its health benefits, I learned to like it. Now I try to eat a cup of broccoli every day, whether I chop it up in a salad, eat it raw with hummus as a snack, or steam it with an entrée for dinner.

An apple a day might keep the doctor away, but eating broccoli every day will do even more for your health. Emerging science suggests that consuming broccoli can alter the way your genes are expressed, thus playing a powerful role in preventing everything from cancer to heart disease. A study of 4,886 breast cancer survivors found a 62 percent reduction in mortality for women whose vegetable consumption was in the highest quartile.

Of all common foods available in the world today, no single food has amassed a body of research about its health benefits that rivals broccoli. It is a rich source of antioxidants, vitamins, and fiber. Research suggests it has powerful anticancer activity and heart benefits, could guard against arthritis and asthma, and helps protect our eyesight and boost our immune system. People are finally taking notice. In one of the most encouraging findings I have read in a long time, per-person consumption of fresh broccoli in the United States has *tripled* over the last three decades.

Find ways to build broccoli and other cruciferous vegetables like cauliflower into your diet. Chop broccoli into small pieces and mix it into a salad or stew. Prepare it with sauces and seasonings that add flavor and taste. Simply steaming fresh broccoli for three to four minutes over medium heat and then adding lemon and pepper is an easy option. If broccoli does not work for you, try kale, bok choy, collard greens, or Swiss chard. There are countless green vegetables you can add to your diet, and all it takes is some creativity to work them into most meals.

Stick With Coffee, Tea, and Water

In liquid form, sugar works in stealth mode. The next time you walk through a grocery store, look at the labels on a few beverages. You will notice the most popular drinks are loaded with added sugars or substitutes.

There are teas with sweeteners that counteract the value of any helpful antioxidants. Many fruit juices have more sugar than you need in an entire week. Even healthy types of milk like almond, coconut, or flax often have added sugars for flavoring. Unless these drinks clearly specify they are "unsweetened," you have to assume they are loaded with additional sugar.

In the United States, about half the population consumes a sugary beverage *every day*, and that is if you *don't* count fruit juice, diet soda, sweetened milk, or sweetened tea. Yet even one to two sugary drinks a day can increase the risk of Type 2 diabetes by more than 25 percent and increase the risk of certain types of cancer. One study found that *each* additional sugar-sweetened drink per day increased the risk of heart disease by 19 percent. A Harvard study estimated sugary drinks alone kill 180,000 people every year.

It appears diet drinks with artificial sweeteners are not much better. The taste of diet drinks makes you crave other sweet foods and may even increase the risk of stroke, depression, and heart attack. For nearly a decade,

I consumed several diet sodas every day. Then as I read more about the detrimental effects of even diet soda and how it could lead me to eat sweeter foods throughout the day, I switched to water, coffee, or tea instead.

I still give in and drink a diet soda on occasion when I'm away from home. Yet what made the most difference for me was never purchasing soda or juice to have at home. As soon as I made that shift and stopped buying diet soda as part of my daily routine at work, I eliminated 98 percent of the problem.

The easiest way to get enough liquid is to drink unlimited quantities of truly natural drinks like coffee, tea, and water. While coffee has received mixed reviews over the years, current research on coffee consumption is over-whelmingly positive. So often, I hear people say, "I need to cut back on coffee." While there are certainly some groups of people who should avoid caffeine, such as expectant mothers, for many people there are tangible benefits to regular coffee consumption.

A study of more than 50,000 women found that two to three cups of caffeinated coffee per day decreased risk of depression by 15 percent, compared with women who had one cup or less per day. Drinking four or more cups helped even more, decreasing the risk of depression by 20 percent.

Emerging research suggests that the high levels of antioxidants in coffee could also help reduce the risk of some cancers. Other studies have shown that coffee can help you live longer, slow down cognitive decline as you age, increase stamina for longer periods of activity, and boost mood. Coffee may also protect against Type 2 diabetes. Some early experiments suggest caffeine's effect on your body mimics the muscle contraction that accompanies exercise.

If you do not tolerate coffee well, tea is a great alternative. It has a quarter of the caffeine of coffee and is easier on the stomach. Green tea in particular offers a host of health benefits, from decreasing inflammation and preventing cancer to protecting your skin. Green tea is also good for your brain, learning, and memory. Just be careful to avoid caffeine in the afternoon or evening so it doesn't disrupt your sleep.

And don't forget to drink lots of water. Hydrating your body flushes toxins from your organs and carries nutrients to your cells. It also provides a moist environment for your ears, nose, and throat, which helps minimize daily irritation. When I have a headache, sinus problems, or allergies, drinking a lot of water often works as well as taking medication.

○ ○ ○

Tame Ties and Tight Pants

Anything you wear that creates discomfort could cause long-term problems. Tight belts can put pressure on critical nerves. Snug-fitting jeans often interfere with digestion and create what one physician dubbed "tight pants syndrome."

Ties and tight collars can limit your movement and decrease circulation to the brain. Ties can even cause eye problems, decreased range of motion in the neck, and increased tension in the back and shoulders. Or as billionaire entrepreneur Richard Branson said far more colorfully in an interview:

"I don't know why the tie was ever invented ... now everyone looks the same and dresses the same. I often have a pair of scissors in my top pocket to go cutting people's ties off. I do think that ties most likely are still inflicted on people because the bosses, they had to wear it for 40 years and when they get into positions of responsibility they're damned if they're going to not have the next generation suffer."

A few years ago, I realized wearing a tie was making me less effective in my job. I was having headaches, skin irritation, and difficulty breathing. But wearing a tie was necessary if I wanted to fit in at important meetings. When I conformed to these unwritten fashion rules, I ended up spending a good deal of time thinking about my own discomfort.

While I was working on this book, my grandmother passed away. Even though I knew I was expected to wear a tie to her funeral service, I decided not to. I wanted to make sure all of my energy was focused on what mattered that day, remembering my grandmother and being there for my family.

If you wear a tie and find it just as comfortable as when you wear an open collar, or if it gives you more confidence, by all means wear one. Women have even more hurdles to deal with. Our society keeps encouraging women to wear high heels and to squeeze into something even smaller each season. There will always be trade-offs and times when a little pain is worth tolerating for an evening. Just make this the exception instead of the norm.

Ill-fitting shoes are another source of daily discomfort that can lead to longer-term problems caused by chronic inflammation. In particular, heels higher than two inches have been linked to a variety of ailments, from stress fractures to shortened Achilles tendons. Find a pair of shoes you can wear for extended periods. There are several shoe brands, for men and women, that specialize in comfortable shoes and look perfectly normal with business apparel.

I am certainly not suggesting you start wearing sweatpants or slippers to work. Looking professional matters in many settings, and you can meet most dress codes without being uncomfortable. After spending the last decade in the business world, I've never seen a meeting fail because someone neglected to wear heels or a tie. Unless you are perfectly comfortable in high heels or ties every day, save these accessories for special events.

○ ○ ○

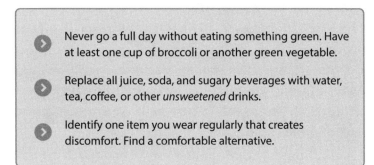

> Never go a full day without eating something green. Have at least one cup of broccoli or another green vegetable.

> Replace all juice, soda, and sugary beverages with water, tea, coffee, or other *unsweetened* drinks.

> Identify one item you wear regularly that creates discomfort. Find a comfortable alternative.

Fight Risk With Food

The greatest risks to your health are specific to you as an individual. This is why doctors ask about your family history and why they collect as much information as possible, from height to weight to blood pressure. Your physician is trying to do what is best based on your individualized risk factors. Yet no doctor will ever have as much insight into your health as you can accumulate.

Your genes, environment, and choices all make unique contributions. Some elements work against you, while others fight back and help. In this constant tug of war, knowledge is your best ally.

Take, for example, my personal condition. Because I was born with a genetic mutation that creates an unusually high risk for cancerous growth, I have a clear understanding of the greatest threats to my health. Armed with this information, I pay close attention to anything related to these vulnerabilities. When I notice a story in the news about something that increases or decreases the odds of kidney cancer, for example, I dig deeper. Several years ago, I saw a headline about a large study that found a relationship between eating fatty fish like salmon and reduction in kidney cancer.

When I tracked down the full report from this study, I discovered that eating just one serving of fatty fish per week was associated with a 44 percent reduction in risk of kidney cancer. The study participants who consumed a serving of fish per week for a decade had a 74 percent decrease in cancer rates. After reading this research, I figured it would not hurt to eat more fatty fish, as long as I selected fish with low mercury levels.

This study was one of many I found related to kidney cancer. Another review found a strong association between increasing BMI (body mass index) and cancer of the kidneys. This work suggests that every one-point increase in BMI increases the risk of kidney cancer by 4 percent. While that may sound small, it translates to a 50 percent higher rate of kidney cancer if you are obese.

These examples are specific to my own risk equation for kidney cancer. Making these small changes will not keep me from developing additional kidney tumors. But in combination with everything else I have learned on these topics, my goal is to reduce my overall risk.

Identify your greatest health risk today, whether it is cancer, heart disease, diabetes, or something more specific. Also consider friends and loved ones who are battling a health condition. Watch news reports for any headlines relating to these risks.

When you spot something with the potential to improve your odds, do some research. Don't change your diet based on unreliable information. If you see something questionable, go to the source and determine if the findings are applicable to your health.

Look for studies that have been published in peer-reviewed medical journals like *The New England Journal of Medicine* (NEJM), *Journal of the American Medical Association* (JAMA), or the *British Medical Journal* (BMJ). The U.S. National Library of Medicine has an enormous database of these articles on its pubmed.gov site, which is available free of charge and a good place to start. Once you have confidence in the source, eat based on what you learn to boost your odds of living longer.

○ ○ ○

Gain Sleep With Weight Loss

The more you weigh, the more difficult it is to get enough sleep. Being overweight or obese is not only a barrier to nighttime sleep, but it also creates daytime sleepiness and lost energy.

Losing weight is one of the best ways to counteract excessive fatigue. But this is clearly a two-way street. Better sleep also helps with weight loss over time. As people's weight goes down and they sleep better, it decreases their risk of other ailments like diabetes, high blood pressure, and heart disease.

If you weigh more than you should today, shedding a few pounds could have a major impact on the quality of your sleep. A Johns Hopkins study found that diet and activity improve sleep quality for people who are overweight. Losing belly fat in particular led to higher quality sleep.

One way to shed pounds is to replace an hour of television with an hour of sleep. This simple change could result in substantial weight loss over time. A study on this topic suggests that swapping this hour of television for sleep could result in a loss of more than 14 pounds over a year.

If you can maintain a lean weight, you will sleep better. Sleeping better, in turn, will decrease your appetite and help you make better dietary choices. Because of the way sleep and diet are closely intertwined, you can create an upward spiral with both elements feeding off one another in a good way. Remember, it starts with your next meal; one day of eating the right foods and a good night's sleep sets a positive cycle in motion.

Eight Is Enough

Think about how many hours you consider to be an ideal night's sleep. Having a clear expectation about how long you want to sleep every night can be a good starting point for improving overall sleep quality. The amount of sleep we need varies from one person to the next. I know people who claim they are at their best as long as they get six good hours of sleep. Others say eight or even nine hours is ideal.

When researchers study the exact amount of sleep people need to feel fully rested, they find that 95 percent of us need somewhere between seven and nine hours of sleep per night. In controlled experiments where subjects are placed in an environment without clocks or windows and asked to sleep when necessary, just 2.5 percent of people (1 in 40) felt well-rested with less than seven hours of sleep a night. Another 2.5 percent needed nine hours or more.

Based on this study and a large body of academic research, it is safe to say the vast majority of people need about eight hours of quality sleep. When scientists test the amount of sleep people need, they use computer programs to track how alert participants are while they conduct on-screen tasks. People who have just seven hours of sleep do not perform as well on these tests compared with participants who sleep more than eight hours.

On the other end of this continuum, people who sleep more than nine hours a night could *increase* their risk of various conditions, from obesity to depression. So the

right range is somewhere between seven and nine hours
of total sleep, depending on your body's unique reaction
to sleep. Most people need seven hours of sleep just to be
in the game the next day and ideally eight to have enough
energy to win.

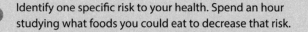

> Identify one specific risk to your health. Spend an hour
studying what foods you could eat to decrease that risk.

> Work toward or maintain a normal weight to improve your
odds of sleeping well. If you need to lose a few pounds,
swap an hour of daily television for an hour of sleep.

> Arrange your schedule to ensure you get at least eight
hours of sleep each night.

Wrapping Up

Every Meal Matters

Every bite and drink counts. The moment you ingest something, it moves through your body, creating positive or negative effects in various places. A donut or sugary drink, for example, creates an immediate high and then does more damage than good by the time it passes through. A leafy green salad, in contrast, functions like a virtual housekeeper as it cleans bad elements from your body and deposits nutrients.

When I was in high school, my biology teacher demonstrated what happens to the human lung as people inhale cigarette smoke. He actually lit a cigarette in our classroom and showed us how the virtual inhaling of smoke created yellowing and browning of a white sponge. It was a powerful visual showing what's happening to your insides when you smoke. Unfortunately, there is no easy way (at least yet) to see the deleterious effects bad dietary choices have inside your body.

Yet, the food and beverages you consume can be just as detrimental as chain smoking. When researchers brought people into a lab and tested the effect of a single poor meal, they made a few surprising discoveries. One group had a healthy meal consisting of salmon, almonds, and vegetables. The researchers conducted an ultrasound of each person's arteries a few hours later. In this group, people's arteries dilated normally (compared to an initial baseline scan) and maintained good blood flow.

A second group was assigned to eat a meal consisting of a sandwich with sausage, egg, and cheese and three hash browns. This group also had baseline ultrasound scans of their arteries and follow-up scans after the bad meal. After eating just one poor meal, the arteries of participants in this group dilated *24 percent less* than their original state. This study suggests *every meal* influences your body's ability to function properly.

Each ounce you consume is either a net positive or a net negative by the time it runs through your body. You don't get healthier by simply trying to eat better in general. You improve your health on a bite-by-bite basis. Once you know what foods and drinks do more good than harm, weigh your choices throughout the day as if you can see the immediate impact of each decision inside your body.

○ ○ ○

Put Activity Before Exercise

How much should you exercise? The scientific answers to this question often conflict with one another based on the type of exercise or whether the study targeted heart disease, weight loss, or a different outcome. Yet there is a simple answer for most of us: *a little more than you are exercising today.*

The thought of "getting in shape" can be overwhelming. The thought of taking a few vigorous steps today is not. When you know you are going to have a day with almost no activity, challenge yourself to get up and take a brisk five-minute walk. Start small. Some activity is always better than none.

The debate about whether you need 30 versus 60 minutes of exercise a day, or five versus six days a week, is more philosophical than practical. If you don't do any formal exercise today, start by walking a few times a week, or spend even 15 minutes engaged in something that increases your heart rate.

One large-scale study suggests that even 15 minutes of activity a day could add three years to your life. Then every additional 15 minutes of activity per day reduces mortality by another 4 percent. The last thing you want to do is set a goal so unrealistic or intimidating that it deters you from doing anything at all. Make sure you don't exercise to the point of creating undue fatigue or soreness, which can keep you from being active the next day.

If you already exercise for 30 minutes two or three days a week, stretch yourself to four and then five days per week. Even when you reach the most common general guideline of 150 minutes of moderate-intensity activity per week, additional activity will continue to help.

Each minute of activity adds up and matters. Experiment with what works best for you. Focus on how you feel, physically and mentally, on days when you are active. See if you notice any patterns, such as better interactions with your friends or additional energy when playing with your children.

Don't just exercise because you "have to" for your physical health. When researchers study the benefits of working out, it clearly does just as much for your mental well-being. In these studies, even a little more exercise can significantly improve your overall satisfaction with life. Added activity has also been shown to provide a physio-logical buffer, so your body does not react as severely to stressful situations throughout the day.

Make a mental note of the immediate return on the time you invest in activity. Use this return on energy and enjoyment to keep going. Build movement into your normal lifestyle so you don't have to worry about "getting in shape" all the time. If you can build on these small wins, a year later, you will notice you also got in shape.

○ ○ ○

Invest in Sleep for Your Future

The better you sleep, the better you eat. Science has shown that good sleep increases your production of the digestive hormone leptin, which keeps you from eating too much. Sound sleep also *decreases* the digestive hormone ghrelin, which boosts appetite.

This could explain why a short night's sleep not only increases hunger, but also causes you to eat calorie-dense high-carbohydrate foods and sweets. When you are in a sleep-deprived state, unhealthy foods activate regions of the brain typically involved in addiction and behavior control. As one researcher described, based on experimental sleep studies conducted in his lab, this could explain our preference for high-fat and high-sugar food when we are tired.

This is another example of how closely intertwined your diet, activity, and sleep patterns are in the span of a day. When you look at some of the leading causes of obesity, it is easy to jump to diet and exercise as a remedy, but sleep clearly belongs in this category. To eat better, make sure your next diet takes the quality of your sleep into account.

When you think about your health, sleep often gets pushed to the back burner. With all the things you need to do in a day, one less hour of sleep seems to be a good way to find extra time. But it is a trap. Sleep is not a luxury. It is a basic necessity.

If you sleep less, you eat more. You remember less. You get sick more often. You look bad. And poor sleep also leads to high blood pressure, missed workouts, irritability, poor decision making, and greatly impaired well-being.

Prioritize eight hours of high-quality sleep ahead of all else. You will be more likely to have a good workout, get more done at your job, and treat your loved ones better when you put sleep first. Remember, every extra hour of sleep is a positive investment. It is not an expense.

○ ○ ○

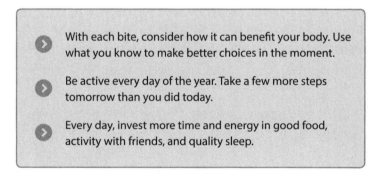

> With each bite, consider how it can benefit your body. Use what you know to make better choices in the moment.

> Be active every day of the year. Take a few more steps tomorrow than you did today.

> Every day, invest more time and energy in good food, activity with friends, and quality sleep.

CONCLUDING THOUGHTS

Putting It All Together

Eat right. Move more. Sleep better. When you do these three things in combination, you will see how the overall benefit is greater than the sum of the parts.

Eating right is not enough. Exercise alone is insufficient. Sleeping well, in isolation, is not adequate. When you focus all your energy on just one of these pursuits, it often comes at the expense of another. It is essential to think about all three elements together.

Eating the right foods provides energy for your workout and improves the quality of your sleep. In turn, a sound night of sleep makes you more likely to eat right the next day. This is why the real magic lies *at the intersection between eating, moving, and sleeping.* If you can do all three well, it will improve your daily energy and your odds of living a long, healthy life.

As I mentioned in the introduction, life itself is a big game of odds. You get to chip away at it, one day at a time. Small decisions and behaviors are quite consequential. In particular, if you have known risks or health conditions today, the way you eat, move, and sleep are the *only things you can control* with each decision.

Once you start to improve your odds of living longer and stronger, take one more step. *Create a culture of health around you.* Rethink everything with this in mind. Leading through example is the single best way to improve the health of the people you love.

Consider how you could fill your home with better foods for yourself and your family. Find a few friends or colleagues who will help you stay active. Create an environment where a sound night's sleep is the norm.

Help yourself. Then help the people you love to live like life depends on it. Because it does.

About the Author

Tom Rath is one of the most influential authors of the last decade. He studies the role of human behavior in health, business, and economics.

Tom has written several international bestsellers, including the #1 *New York Times* bestseller *How Full Is Your Bucket?* In 2012, his book *StrengthsFinder 2.0* was the top-selling nonfiction book worldwide. Tom's most recent *New York Times* bestsellers are *Strengths Based Leadership* and *Wellbeing: The Five Essential Elements*. In total, his books have sold more than 5 million copies and have made more than 250 appearances on the *Wall Street Journal* bestseller list.

Tom serves as a senior scientist and advisor to Gallup, where he previously spent 13 years leading the organization's work on employee engagement, strengths, and well-being. Tom also served as vice chairman of the VHL cancer research organization. He earned degrees from the University of Michigan and the University of Pennsylvania, where he is now a guest lecturer. Tom and his wife, Ashley, and their two children live in Arlington, Virginia.

More information:

Website: www.tomrath.org
Twitter: @TomCRath
Email: tom@tomrath.org
LinkedIn: www.linkedin.com/in/trath
Facebook: www.facebook.com/authortomrath

EAT MOVE SLEEP

First 30 Days Challenge

DAY 1: The Basics

☐ Identify the healthiest elements of diets you have tried. Build them in to your lifestyle for good.

☐ Each morning, plan ahead to add activity to your daily routine.

☐ Sleep longer tonight to do more tomorrow.

DAY 2: Small Adjustments

☐ Ask yourself if the next food you put in your mouth is a net gain or a net loss. Repeat throughout the day.

☐ Eliminate an hour of chair time from your daily routine.

☐ Gradually add sleep to your nightly schedule in 15-minute increments. Continue until you feel fully rested each morning.

DAY 3: Quality First

☐ Select one food to eat today with a balanced (1 to 1) ratio of carbs to protein. Avoid foods above a ratio of 5 to 1.

☐ Put the healthiest foods in your home on a shelf at eye level or in a bowl on the counter.

☐ Identify one way you can work *without* sitting, right now. Test it out tomorrow.

DAY 4: Break The Cycle

☐ Identify the sugar content in your favorite meal or snack. If it's more than 10g, find a replacement.

☐ Pick one food or drink you sweeten regularly — artificially or with sugar — and consume it without the added sweetener for a week.

☐ When you have to sit for long periods of time, stand up, walk, or stretch every 20 minutes.

DAY 5: Staying Healthy

☐ Every time you go to the store, start by loading up on fruits and vegetables with vibrant colors.

☐ When disruptions threaten your regular schedule, plan ahead to ensure you get a good night's sleep.

☐ As you make adjustments for better sleep, measure your progress. Note the time you get into bed and the time you wake up. Then rate your sleep quality on a 1-10 scale.

DAY 6: What Counts

☐ Build your meals around fruits and vegetables today to change the expression of your genes tomorrow.

☐ Select one way to measure your daily movement. Use a pedometer, watch, GPS, smartphone, or manual log to start tracking your activity today.

☐ Aim for 10,000 steps every day or 70,000 steps per week.

DAY 7: Refined Fuel

- [ ] Replace chips, crackers, and snack bars with nuts, seeds, apples, celery, and carrots.
- [ ] Always leave the serving dishes in the kitchen; don't bring them to the table.
- [ ] Get a full hour of vigorous activity to burn calories all day long.

DAY 8: Timing Matters

- [ ] Select a healthy standby snack today. Carry it with you wherever you go.
- [ ] Make every meal last at least 20 minutes.
- [ ] Exercise in the morning for a better mood and more brainpower all day.

DAY 9: Shortcuts

- [ ] Make a healthy choice and order first when you dine out. It will lock in your good decision and likely start a trend.
- [ ] Pick one of your most repetitive motions, such as using a smartphone, computer, or carrying a heavy bag. Alternate use of your left and right sides frequently.
- [ ] Use bright light to stay alert during the day. Dim your lights in the evening. Then block all light in your bedroom at night.

DAY 10: Decisions

☐ Investigate how you can get most of your protein from plant-based sources.

☐ Quit giving people food you know better than to eat yourself. When buying food for friends or preparing a meal for others, think of what's best for their health.

☐ Pick one deeply personal motivation to move more. Find a way to remind yourself every day with a photo, note, or quote.

DAY 11: Working

☐ Engineer activity into your work. Have a standing or walking meeting. Get up and move every time you are on the phone.

☐ Take a midday break of at least 30 minutes every day.

☐ Structure your work schedule for better sleep. Help your boss and colleagues understand why good sleep is in everyone's best interest.

DAY 12: Quitting

☐ Whenever you receive junk food, put it in the nearest trash can. This will keep you from splurging or regifting it.

☐ When you see a friend making a good decision about what to eat, give credit and encouragement.

☐ Avoid using the snooze button on your alarm for the next week. Then, see if you can banish it for good.

DAY 13: Myth Busting

- [ ] When you are offered complimentary bread with a meal, ask for a healthy alternative or simply pass.

- [ ] Eliminate one type of red or processed meat from your diet for good (like bacon or hot dogs).

- [ ] Keep your bedroom two to four degrees cooler at night. See if it helps you fall asleep and stay asleep.

DAY 14: Home

- [ ] Use smaller cups, plates, and serving sizes to eat less.

- [ ] Identify one easy way to add activity around your home or neighborhood: walking, running, biking, exercise machines, workout videos, yoga, or Pilates.

- [ ] Discuss how schedules, lighting, thermostats, and reducing noise can help everyone living under your roof sleep better.

DAY 15: Get Ahead

- [ ] Select restaurants based on how easy it is to make a healthy choice when you order.

- [ ] When you are tempted to skip a workout, just start exercising for a few minutes. Starting is often the hardest part.

- [ ] The next time you work on something that requires a great deal of learning and synthesizing, go to bed early instead of staying up late.

DAY 16: Energy

☐ Before you order a heavy lunch, consider whether you can afford the hangover that afternoon.

☐ When your brain is filled with new information to remember or when you need a burst of creativity, go for a walk.

☐ If you're having trouble sleeping, try exercising for a few days before you resort to sleep medication.

DAY 17: Expectations

☐ Pick one food you eat even though you know you shouldn't. Give it an entertaining nickname that will make you think twice about eating it.

☐ Shop for foods based on whether they are good for you first. Then consider buying organic if you eat the skin.

☐ Identify a specific goal for increasing your activity. Write it down, add a deadline, and share it with at least one person (ideally more) or post it online.

DAY 18: Good Nights

☐ Structure your days to eat more early, less late, and nothing after dinner.

☐ Limit yourself to two hours of *seated* television a day.

☐ Create a routine so you don't eat, drink, or use electronic messaging in the hour before you go to bed.

DAY 19: Think Again

- [ ] Replace all dried fruits and fruit juices with whole fruit and other healthy alternatives.

- [ ] If you see a packaged food or drink claiming to be healthy on the surface, study all the ingredients in even more detail.

- [ ] If sounds wake you up at night, add a constant background noise to keep them from interrupting your sleep. Try a fan, noisemaker, or smartphone app.

DAY 20: Your Routine

- [ ] Steam healthy foods like fish and vegetables instead of grilling them with dry heat.

- [ ] Find one way to trim your total weekly transit time, like telecommuting once a week or driving at low-traffic times.

- [ ] Wake up at the same general time every day of the week to keep your internal clock on track.

DAY 21: Simple Steps

- [ ] Go through the food in your house today. Get rid of a few unhealthy items that have been sitting on a shelf for months.

- [ ] If you are in motion, whether walking or driving, keep your smartphone in your pocket or purse.

- [ ] Identify one thing that stresses you out regularly. Create a plan to prevent it from occurring in the first place.

DAY 22: Looking Good

☐ Eat more carrots and tomatoes for a truly natural tan. Also add salmon and blueberries for better hair and skin.

☐ Walk at least five minutes a day to counteract aging. Build up to 45 minutes of intense activity at least three days a week to halt aging even more.

☐ When you need to look your best, give yourself plenty of time to get a sound night's sleep.

DAY 23: An Extra Boost

☐ Start every meal with the *most* healthy item on your plate, and end with the *least*.

☐ Identify one aerobic activity that gives you a natural high. Do it at least once a week for 30 minutes.

☐ At the end of a lousy day, before you make a small stressor into something bigger, give sleep a chance to do some repair work overnight.

DAY 24: Reminders

☐ When you want a quick snack, take a handful and leave the bag or box behind.

☐ Spend at least five minutes outside every day.

☐ Identify one person who will check in regularly and hold you accountable for staying active. This could be a friend, coach, or personal trainer.

DAY 25: Prevention

☐ Replace sweet and fried foods with healthier spices and flavors.

☐ Make activity your first line of defense before you resort to pain killers or other medications.

☐ Know your blood pressure and cholesterol levels. If you don't know these numbers, check them in the next month. Then retest at least once per year.

DAY 26: Daily Choices

☐ Identify a few healthy food options. Buy them automatically so good choices are always available at home.

☐ Use vigorous exercise to clear your mind and body.

☐ Make small decisions quickly to get them out of the way. But when you need to make a big decision, always sleep on it first.

DAY 27: New Habits

☐ Save sugary desserts for *your own* birthday. On other occasions, eat fruit or berries instead.

☐ Ration your most indulgent choices to enjoy them even more. If you can't imagine life without chocolate, have a few bites once a week.

☐ Try a new microactivity today, like taking the stairs or parking far away from the door.

DAY 28: Trend Setters

☐ Never go a full day without eating something green. Have at least one cup of broccoli or another green vegetable.

☐ Replace all juice, soda, and sugary beverages with water, tea, coffee, or other *unsweetened* drinks.

☐ Identify one item you wear regularly that creates discomfort. Find a comfortable alternative.

DAY 29: Ideas for Life

☐ Identify one specific risk to your health. Spend an hour studying what foods you could eat to decrease that risk.

☐ Work toward or maintain a normal weight to improve your odds of sleeping well. If you need to lose a few pounds, swap an hour of daily television for an hour of sleep.

☐ Arrange your schedule to ensure you get at least eight hours of sleep each night.

DAY 30: Wrapping Up

☐ With each bite, consider how it can benefit your body. Use what you know to make better choices in the moment.

☐ Be active every day of the year. Take a few more steps tomorrow than you did today.

☐ Every day, invest more time and energy in good food, activity with friends, and quality sleep.

Notes

As I mentioned in the book's opening, there is an extraordinary amount of high-quality research available today to help us lead longer and healthier lives. Almost all of the content in this book rests on the shoulders of doctors, clinical researchers, and other writers who have helped share these discoveries with the world.

I highly encourage you to use the interactive **Reference Explorer** at **www.eatmovesleep.org** to dive into the areas that interest you most throughout the book. These sections will be updated regularly on the website as new findings emerge. To find a direct link to any of the following articles on the website, *note the corresponding number (1 through 408) to the left of each article* on the following pages.

Introduction

1. Jones, D. S., Podolsky, S. H., & Greene, J. A. (2012). The burden of disease and the changing task of medicine. *New England Journal of Medicine, 366*(25), 2333–2338. doi:10.1056/NEJMp1113569
2. VHL.org. (2013, March 02). Basic facts about VHL. Retrieved from http://www.vhl.org/patients-caregivers/basic-facts-about-vhl/
3. Simple lifestyle changes can add a decade or more healthy years to the average lifespan, Canadian study shows. (2011, October 21). *ScienceDaily*. Retrieved from http://www.sciencedaily.com/releases/2011/10/111021074730.htm
4. Lifestyle affects life expectancy more than genetics, Swedish study finds. (2011, February 8). *ScienceDaily*. Retrieved from http://www.sciencedaily.com/releases/2011/02/110207112539.htm
5. Wilhelmsen, L., Svärdsudd, K., Eriksson, H., Rosengren, A., Hansson, P.-O., Welin, C., Odén, A., & Welin, L. (2011). Factors associated with reaching 90 years of age: A study of men born in 1913 in Gothenburg, Sweden. *Journal of Internal Medicine, 269*(4), 441–451. doi:10.1111/j.1365-2796.2010.02331.x
6. King A. C., Castro, C. M., Buman, M. P., Hekler, E. B., Urizar, G. G., & Ahn, D. K. (2013). Behavioral impacts of sequentially versus simultaneously delivered dietary plus physical activity interventions: The CALM Trial. *Annals of Behavioral Medicine*. doi: 10.1007/s12160-013-9501-y

Chapter One

7. The International Food Information Council (2012, May). Americans find doing their own taxes simpler than improving diet and health. Retrieved June 5, 2013, from http://www.foodinsight.org/Content/3840/FINAL 2012 Food and Health Exec Summary.pdf
8. Centers for Disease Control (n.d.). FastStats: Obesity and overweight. Retrieved June 5, 2013, from http://www.cdc.gov/nchs/fastats/overwt.htm
9. Ebbeling C.B., Swain, J. F., Feldman, H. A., Wong, W. W., Hachey, D. L., GarciaLago, E., & Ludwig, D. S. (2012). Effects of dietary composition on energy expenditure during weight-loss maintenance. *Journal of the American Medical Association, 307*(24), 2627–2634. doi:10.1001/jama.2012.6607
10. Mooney, A. (2012). When a calorie is not just a calorie. *Harvard Gazette*. Retrieved March 6, 2013, from http://news.harvard.edu/gazette/story/2012/06/when-a-calorie-is-not-just-a-calorie/

11. Mozaffarian, D., Hao, T., Rimm, E. B., Willett, W. C., & Hu, F. B. (2011). Changes in diet and lifestyle and long-term weight gain in women and men. *New England Journal of Medicine, 364*(25), 2392-2404. doi:10.1056/NEJMoa1014296

12. Brody, J. E. (2011, July 18). Still counting calories? Your weight-loss plan may be outdated. *The New York Times*. Retrieved from http://www.nytimes.com/2011/07/19/health/19brody.html?pagewanted=all&_r=1&

13. Dreifus, C. (2012, May 14). A mathematical challenge to obesity. *The New York Times*. Retrieved from http://www.nytimes.com/2012/05/15/science/a-mathematical-challenge-to-obesity.html

14. Owen, N., Bauman, A., & Brown, W. (2009). Too much sitting: A novel and important predictor of chronic disease risk? *British Journal of Sports Medicine, 43*(2), 81–83. doi:10.1136/bjsm.2008.055269

15. Vlahos, J. (2011, April 14). Is sitting a lethal activity? *The New York Times Magazine*. Retrieved from http://www.nytimes.com/2011/04/17/magazine/mag-17sitting-t.html

16. Thorp, A. A., Owen, N., Neuhaus, M., & Dunstan, D. W. (2011). Sedentary behaviors and subsequent health outcomes in adults: A systematic review of longitudinal studies, 1996-2011. *American Journal of Preventive Medicine, 41*(2), 207–215. doi:10.1016/j.amepre.2011.05.004

17. Matthews, C. E., George, S. M., Moore, S. C., Bowles, H. R., Blair, A., Park, Y., Troiano, R. P., & Schatzkin, A. (2012). Amount of time spent in sedentary behaviors and cause-specific mortality in US adults. *American Journal of Clinical Nutrition, 95*(2), 437–445. doi:10.3945/ajcn.111.019620

18. Patel, A. V., Bernstein, L., Deka, A., Feigelson, H. S., Campbell, P. T., Gapstur, S. M., Colditz, G. A., & Thun, M. J. (2010). Leisure time spent sitting in relation to total mortality in a prospective cohort of US adults. *American Journal of Epidemiology, 172*(4), 419–429. doi:10.1093/aje/kwq155

19. Fryer, B. (2006). Sleep deficit: The performance killer. *Harvard Business Review*. Retrieved June 5, 2013, from http://hbr.org/2006/10/sleep-deficit-the-performance-killer/ar/1#

20. Ericsson, K. A., Krampe, R. T., & Tesch-Römer, C. (1993). The role of deliberate practice in the acquisition of expert performance. *Psychological Review, 100*(3), 363–406. doi:10.1037/0033-295X.100.3.363

21. National Sleep Foundation. (2013). National Sleep Foundation poll finds exercise key to good sleep. Retrieved March 6, 2013, from http://www.sleepfoundation.org/alert/national-sleep-foundation-poll-finds-exercise-key-good-sleep

22. Sluckhaupt, S. E. (2012). Short sleep duration among workers: United States, 2010. *Morbidity & Mortality Weekly Report, 61*(16), 281-285. Retrieved June 5, 2013, from http://www.cdc.gov/mmwr/pdf/wk/mm6116.pdf

23. Rosekind, M. R., Gregory, K. B., Mallis, M. M., Brandt, S. L., Seal, B., & Lerner, D. (2010). The cost of poor sleep: Workplace productivity loss and associated costs. *Journal of Occupational and Environmental Medicine, 52*(1), 91–98. doi:10.1097/JOM.0b013e3181c78c30

24. Söderström, M., Jeding, K., Ekstedt, M., Perski, A., & Åkerstedt, T. (2012). Insufficient sleep predicts clinical burnout. *Journal of Occupational Health Psychology, 17*(2), 175-183.

25. Schwartz, T. (2013, February 9). Relax! You'll be more productive. *The New York Times*. Retrieved from http://www.nytimes.com/2013/02/10/opinion/sunday/relax-youll-be-more-productive.html

Chapter Two

26. Rath, T. & Harter, J. K. (2010). *Wellbeing: The five essential elements*. New York: Gallup Press.

27. Lee, I.-M., Shiroma, E. J., Lobelo, F., Puska, P., Blair, S. N., & Katzmarzyk, P. T. (2012). Effect of physical inactivity on major non-communicable diseases worldwide: An analysis of burden of disease and life expectancy. *The Lancet, 380*(9838), 219–229. doi:10.1016/S0140-6736(12)61031-9

28. Patel, A. V., Bernstein, L., Deka, A., Feigelson, H. S., Campbell, P. T., Gapstur, S. M., Colditz, G. A., & Thun, M. J. (2010). Leisure time spent sitting in relation to total mortality in a prospective cohort of US adults. *American Journal of Epidemiology, 172*(4), 419–429. doi:10.1093/aje/kwq155

29. Granados, K., Stephens, B. R., Malin, S. K., Zderic, T. W., Hamilton, M. T., & Braun, B. (2012). Appetite regulation in response to sitting and energy imbalance. *Applied Physiology, Nutrition, and Metabolism, 37*(2), 323–333. doi:10.1139/h2012-002

30. Sitting is killing you. (n.d.). In *Medical Billing and Coding Certification.* Retrieved July 1, 2013 from http://www.medicalbillingandcoding.org/sitting-kills/

31. Sitting at a desk all day is 'as bad for health as smoking.' (2007). In *Mail Online.* Retrieved June 5, 2013, from http://www.dailymail.co.uk/news/article-492543/Sitting-desk-day-bad-health-smoking.html

32. Hamilton, M. T., Hamilton, R. G., & Zderic, T. W. (2007). Role of low energy expenditure and sitting in obesity, metabolic syndrome, type 2 diabetes, and cardiovascular disease. *Diabetes, 56,* 2655-2666.

33. Hellmich, N. (2012, August 13). Take a stand against sitting disease. *USA Today.* Retrieved from http://www.usatoday.com/news/health/story/2012-07-19/sitting-disease-questions-answers/57016756/1

34. Sitting is killing you. (n.d.). In *Medical Billing and Coding Certification.* Retrieved July 1, 2013 from http://www.medicalbillingandcoding.org/sitting-kills/

35. Sitting at a desk all day is 'as bad for health as smoking.' (2007). In *Mail Online.* Retrieved June 5, 2013, from http://www.dailymail.co.uk/news/article-492543/Sitting-desk-day-bad-health-smoking.html

36. National Sleep Foundation. (2013, March 4). National Sleep Foundation poll finds exercise key to good sleep. Retrieved from http://www.sleepfoundation.org/alert/national-sleep-foundation-poll-finds-exercise-key-good-sleep

37. Manber, R., Bootzin, R. R., Acebo, C., & Carskadon, M. A. (1996). The effects of regularizing sleep-wake schedules on daytime sleepiness. *Sleep, 19*(5), 432–441.

38. Agus, D. B. (2011). *The end of illness.* New York: Free Press.

Chapter Three

39. Melnick, M. (2011, October 24). Study: Why people don't read nutrition labels. *Time.* Retrieved from http://healthland.time.com/2011/10/24/study-why-people-dont-read-nutrition-labels/

40. Graham, D. J., & Jeffery, R. W. (2011). Location, location, location: Eye-tracking evidence that consumers preferentially view prominently positioned nutrition information. *Journal of the American Dietetic Association, 111*(11), 1704–1711. doi:10.1016/j.jada.2011.08.005

41. Larsen, T. M., Dalskov, S. M., van Baak, M., Jebb, S. A., Papadaki, A., Pfeiffer, A. F., Martinez, J. A., Handjieva-Darlenska, T., Kunešová, M., Pihlsgård, M., Stender, S., Holst, C., Sarish, W. H., & Astrup, A. (2010). Diets with high or low protein content and glycemic index for weight-loss maintenance. *New England Journal of Medicine, 363*(22), 2102-2113. doi:10.1056/NEJMoa1007137

42. Hannley, P. P. (2012). Back to the future: Rethinking the way we eat. *American Journal of Medicine, 125*(10), 947–948. doi:10.1016/j.amjmed.2012.07.012

43. Boyle, T., Fritschi, L., Heyworth, J., & Bull, F. (2011). Long-term sedentary work and the risk of subsite-specific colorectal cancer. *American Journal of Epidemiology, 173*(10), 1183–1191. doi:10.1093/aje/kwq513

44. LifeSpan TR1200-DT Treadmill Desk. (2013). LifeSpan Fitness.

45. FitDesk Semi-Recumbent Pedal Desk. (2012). FitDesk.
46. Stafford, P. (2012, April 24). Report claims sitting down is bad for business: Here are three solutions. *SmartCompany*. Retrieved from http://www.smartcompany.com.au/managing-people/049345-sitting-down-is-bad-for-business-report.html

Chapter Four

47. Taubes, G. (2011, April 13). Is sugar toxic? *The New York Times Magazine*. Retrieved from http://www.nytimes.com/2011/04/17/magazine/mag-17Sugar-t.html
48. USDA Office of Communications. (2013, March 02). Chapter 2: Profiling food consumption on America. In *Agricultural Fact Book 2001-2002*. Retrieved June 5, 2013, from http://www.usda.gov/factbook/chapter2.htm
49. UNODC, World Drug Report 2010 (United Nations Publications, sales No. E.10.XI.13). https://www.unodc.org/documents/wdr/WDR_2010/World_Drug_Report_2010_lo-res.pdf
50. Wade, L. (2013, March 19). Sugary drinks linked to 180,000 deaths worldwide. *CNN*. Retrieved from http://www.cnn.com/2013/03/19/health/sugary-drinks-deaths/index.html
51. Centers for Disease Control and Prevention (2012, January 13). Prescription drug overdoses — a U.S. epidemic. *CDC Grand Rounds, 61*(1), 10-13. Retrieved from http://www.cdc.gov/mmwr/preview/mmwrhtml/mm6101a3.htm
52. Simple sugar, lactate, is like 'candy for cancer cells': Cancer cells accelerate aging and inflammation in the body to drive tumor growth. (2011, May 28). *ScienceDaily*. Retrieved from http://www.sciencedaily.com /releases/2011/05/110526152549.htm
53. Liu, H., Huang, D., McArthur, D. L., Boros, L. G., Nissen, N., & Heaney, A. P. (2010). Fructose induces transketolase flux to promote pancreatic cancer growth. *Cancer Research, 70*(15), 6368–6376. doi:10.1158/0008-5472.CAN-09-4615
54. Excess sugar linked to cancer. (2013, Februrary 1). *ScienceDaily*. Retrieved from http://www.sciencedaily.com/releases/2013/02/130201100149.htm
55. Cherbuin, N., Sachdev, P., & Anstey, K. J. (2012). Higher normal fasting plasma glucose is associated with hippocampal atrophy: The PATH Study. *Neurology, 79*(10), 1019–1026. doi:10.1212/WNL.0b013e31826846de
56. Theiss, E. (2010, October 11). Our brains are built to love sugar, thanks to feel-good chemical dopamine. *The Plain Dealer Extra*. [Web log]. Retrieved from http://blog.cleveland.com/pdextra/2010/10/our_brains_are_built_to_love_s.html
57. Laying bare the not-so-sweet tale of a sugar and its role in the spread of cancer. (2011, April 25). *ScienceDaily*. Retrieved from http://www.sciencedaily.com /releases/2011/04/110425120346.htm
58. Yin, X., Johns, S. C., Lawrence, R., Xu, D., Reddi, K., Bishop, J. R., Varner, J. A., & Fuster, M. M. (2011). Lymphatic endothelial heparan sulfate deficiency results in altered growth responses to vascular endothelial growth factor-C (VEGF-C). *Journal of Biological Chemistry, 286*(17), 14952–14962. doi:10.1074/jbc.M110.206664
59. American Heart Association (2013, May 6). Sugars and Carbohydrates. Retrieved from http://www.heart.org/HEARTORG/GettingHealthy/NutritionCenter/Healthy-DietGoals/Sugars-and-Carbohydrates_UCM_303296_Article.jsp
60. Dailey, K. (2009, June 25). The sweet science: How our brain reacts to sugary tastes. *The Daily Beast*. [Web log]. Retrieved from http://www.thedailybeast.com/newsweek/blogs/the-human-condition/2009/06/25/the-sweet-science-how-our-brain-reacts-to-sugary-tastes.html
61. Strawbridge, H. (2012, July 16). Artificial sweeteners: Sugar-free, but at what cost? *Harvard Health Blog*. [Web log]. Retrieved from http://www.health.harvard.edu/blog/artificial-sweeteners-sugar-free-but-at-what-cost-201207165030

62. Fowler, S. P., Williams, K., Resendez, R. G., Hunt, K. J., Hazuda, H. P., & Stern, M. P. (2008). Fueling the obesity epidemic? Artificially sweetened beverage use and long-term weight gain. *Obesity, 16*(8), 1894–1900. doi:10.1038/oby.2008.284

63. CBS News. (2012, April 1). Is sugar toxic? [Video file]. Retrieved from http://www.cbsnews.com/video/watch/?id=7403942n&tag=api Timecode 6:00

64. Stanhope, K. L., Bremer, A. A., Medici, V., Nakajima, K., Ito, Y., Nakano, T., Chen, G., Fong, T. H., Menorca, R. I., Keim, N. L., & Havel, P. J. (2011). Consumption of fructose and high fructose corn syrup increase postprandial Triglycerides, LDL-cholesterol, and apolipoprotein-B in young men and women. *Journal of Clinical Endocrinology & Metabolism, 96*(10), E1596-1605. doi:10.1210/jc.2011-1251

65. Hazell, K. (2011, May 12). Sitting down makes your bottom bigger, study reveals. *The Huffington Post.* Retrieved from http://www.huffingtonpost.co.uk/2011/12/05/sitting-down-makes-your-bottom-bigger-say-experts_n_1129377.html

66. Shoham, N., Gottlieb, R., Shaharabani-Yosef, O., Zaretsky, U., Benayahu, D., & Gefen, A. (2011). Static mechanical stretching accelerates lipid production in 3T3-L1 adipocytes by activating the MEK signaling pathway. *American Journal of Cell Physiology, 302*(2), C429-441. doi:10.1152/ajpcell.00167.2011

67. Dunstan, D. W., Kingwell, B. A., Larsen, R., Healy, G. N., Cerin, E., Hamilton, M. T., Shaw, J. E., Bertovic, D. A., Zimmet, P. Z., Salmon, J., & Owen, N. (2012). Breaking up prolonged sitting reduces postprandial glucose and insulin responses. *Diabetes Care, 35*(5), 976–983. doi:10.2337/dc11-1931

68. Ariga, A., & Lleras, A. (2011). Brief and rare mental "breaks" keep you focused: Deactivation and reactivation of task goals preempt vigilance decrements. *Cognition, 118*(3), 439–443. doi:10.1016/j.cognition.2010.12.007

69. Korkki, P. (2012, June 16). To stay on schedule, take a break. *The New York Times.* Retrieved from http://www.nytimes.com/2012/06/17/jobs/take-breaks-regularly-to-stay-on-schedule-workstation.html

Chapter Five

70. Li, C., Ford, E. S., Zhao, G., Balluz, L. S., Giles, W. H., & Liu, S. (2011). Serum {alpha}-carotene concentrations and risk of death among US adults: The third National Health and Nutrition Examination Survey follow-up study. *Archives of Internal Medicine, 171*(6), 507–515. doi:10.1001/archinternmed.2010.440

71. Blanchflower, D. G., Oswald, A. J., & Stewart-Brown, S. (2012). Is psychological well-being linked to the consumption of fruit and vegetables? (Working Paper No. 18469). *National Bureau of Economic Research.* Retrieved from http://www.nber.org/papers/w18469

72. Diverse diet of veggies may decrease lung cancer risk. (2010, August 31). *ScienceDaily.* Retrieved from http://www.sciencedaily.com /releases/2010/08/100831134822.htm

73. Peng, C., Chan, H. Y. E., Huang, Y., Yu, H., & Chen, Z.-Y. (2011). Apple polyphenols extend the mean lifespan of Drosophila melanogaster. *Journal of Agricultural and Food Chemistry, 59*(5), 2097–2106. doi:10.1021/jf1046267

74. Kell, D. B. (2010). Towards a unifying, systems biology understanding of large-scale cellular death and destruction caused by poorly liganded iron: Parkinson's, Huntington's, Alzheimer's, prions, bactericides, chemical toxicology and others as examples. *Archives of Toxicology, 84*(11), 825–889. doi:10.1007/s00204-010-0577-x

75. Burton-Freeman, B., & Reimers, K. (2011). Tomato consumption and health: Emerging benefits. *American Journal of Lifestyle Medicine, 5*(2), 182–191. doi:10.1177/1559827610387488

76. Cohen, S., Doyle, W. J., Alper, C. M., Janicki-Deverts, D., & Turner, R. B. (2009). Sleep habits and susceptibility to the common cold. *Archives of Internal Medicine, 169*(1), 62–67. doi:10.1001/archinternmed.2008.505

77. Fung, M. M., Peters, K., Redline, S., Ziegler, M. G., Ancoli-Israel, S., Barrett-Connor, E., & Stone, K. L. (2011). Decreased slow wave sleep increases risk of developing hypertension in elderly men. *Hypertension, 58*(4), 596–603. doi:10.1161/ HYPERTENSIONAHA.111.174409

78. Poor sleep quality increases inflammation, community study finds. (2010, November 14). *ScienceDaily.* Retrieved from http://www.sciencedaily.com / releases/2010/11/101114161939.htm

79. Cappuccio, F. P., Cooper, D., D'Elia, L., Strazzullo, P., & Miller, M. A. (2011). Sleep duration predicts cardiovascular outcomes: A systematic review and meta-analysis of prospective studies. *European Heart Journal, 32*(12), 1484–1492. doi:10.1093/eurheartj/ ehr007

80. Cohen, S., Doyle, W. J., Alper, C. M., Janicki-Deverts, D., & Turner, R. B. (2009). Sleep habits and susceptibility to the common cold. *Archives of Internal Medicine, 169*(1), 62–67. doi:10.1001/archinternmed.2008.505

Chapter Six

81. Li, S., Zhao, J. H., Luan, J., Ekelund, U., Luben, R. N., Khaw, K.-T., Wareham, N. J., & Loos, R. J. F. (2010). Physical activity attenuates the genetic predisposition to obesity in 20,000 men and women from EPIC-Norfolk Prospective Population Study. *PLoS Med, 7*(8), e1000332. doi:10.1371/journal.pmed.1000332

82. Ornish, D., Magbanua, M. J. M., Weidner, G., Weinberg, V., Kemp, C., Green, C., Mattie, M. D., Simko, J., Shinohara, K., Hagg, C. M., & Carroll, P. R. (2008). Changes in prostate gene expression in men undergoing an intensive nutrition and lifestyle intervention. *Proceedings of the National Academy of Sciences, 105*(24), 8369–8374. doi:10.1073/ pnas.0803080105

83. Dunham, W. (2008, June 18). Healthy lifestyle triggers genetic changes: Study. *Reuters.* Retrieved from http://www.reuters.com/article/2008/06/18/ us-genes-lifestyle-idUSN1628897920080618

84. Do, R., Xie, C., Zhang, X., Männistö, S., Harald, K., Islam, S., Bailey, S. D., Rangarajan, S., McQueen, M. J., Diaz, R., Lisheng, L., Wang, X., Silander, K., Peltonen, L., Yusuf, S., Salomaa, V., Engert, J. C., & Anand, S. S. (2011). The effect of chromosome 9p21 variants on cardiovascular disease may be modified by dietary intake: Evidence from a case/control and a prospective study. *PLoS Med, 8*(10), e1001106. doi:10.1371/journal. pmed.1001106

85. Bravata, D. M., Smith-Spangler, C., Sundaram, V., Gienger, A. L., Lin, N., Lewis, R., Stave, C. D., Olkin, I., & Sirard, J. R. (2007). Using pedometers to increase physical activity and improve health: A systematic review. *Journal of the American Medical Association, 298*(19), 2296–2304. doi:10.1001/jama.298.19.2296

86. Bassett, D. R., Wyatt, H. R., Thompson, H., Peters, J. C., & Hill, J. O. (2010). Pedometer-measured physical activity and health behaviors in U.S. adults. *Medicine & Science in Sports & Exercise, 42*(10), 1819–1825. doi:10.1249/MSS.0b013e3181dc2e54

87. Lloyd, J. (2010, October 4). Walk this way: U.S. out of step with weight loss. *USA Today.* Retrieved from http://usatoday30.usatoday.com/yourlife/fitness/2010-10-05-walking05_ST_N.htm?csp=usat.me

88. Dwyer, T., Ponsonby, A. L., Ukoumunne, O. C., Pezic, A., Venn, A., Dunstan, D., Barr, E., Blair, S., Cochrane, J., Zimmet, P., & Shaw, J. (2011). Association of change in daily step count over five years with insulin sensitivity and adiposity: population based cohort study. *British Medical Journal, 342*, c7249–c7249. doi:10.1136/ bmj.c7249

Chapter Seven

89. Jameson, M. (2010, December 20). A reversal on carbs. *Los Angeles Times.* Retrieved from http://articles.latimes.com/2010/dec/20/health/la-he-carbs-20101220

90. Scott, P. J. (2011, March). Are carbs more addictive than cocaine? *Details*. Retrieved from http://www.details.com/style-advice/the-body/201103/carbs-caffeine-food-cocaine-addiction

91. Mozaffarian, D., & Ludwig, D. S. (2010). Dietary guidelines in the 21st century—a time for food. *Journal of the American Medical Association, 304*(6), 681–682. doi:10.1001/jama.2010.1116

92. Ho, V. W., Leung, K., Hsu, A., Luk, B., Lai, J., Shen, S. Y., Minchinton, A. I., Waterhouse, D., Bally, M. B., Lin, W., Nelson, B. H., Sly, L. M., & Krystal, G. (2011). A low carbohydrate, high protein diet slows tumor growth and prevents cancer initiation. *Cancer Research, 71*(13), 4484–4493. doi:10.1158/0008-5472.CAN-10-3973

93. Ren, X., Ferreira, J. G., Zhou, L., Shammah-Lagnado, S. J., Yeckel, C. W., & De Araujo, I. E. (2010). Nutrient selection in the absence of taste receptor signaling. *Journal of Neuroscience, 30*(23), 8012–8023. doi:10.1523/JNEUROSCI.5749-09.2010

94. Payne, C., Smith, L., Lee, J., & Wansink, B. (n.d.). Serve it here; eat it there: Serving off the stove results in less food intake than serving off the table. Retrieved March 3, 2013, from http://foodpsychology.cornell.edu/images/posters/serveofftable.pdf

95. Knab, A. M., Shanley, R. A., Corbin, K., Jin, F., Sha, W., & Nieman, D. C. (2011). A 45-minute vigorous exercise bout increases metabolic rate for 19 hours. *Medicine & Science in Sports & Exercise, 43*(9), 1643-1648. doi:10.1249/MSS.0b013e3182118891.

Chapter Eight

96. Page, K. A., Seo, D., Belfort-DeAguiar, R., Lacadie, C., Dzuira, J., Naik, S., Amarnath, S., Sherwin, R. S., & Sinha, R. (2011). Circulating glucose levels modulate neural control of desire for high-calorie foods in humans. *Journal of Clinical Investigation, 121*(10), 4161–4169. doi:10.1172/JCI57873

97. Wansink B., Aner, T., & Shimzu, M. (2012). First foods most: After 18-hour fast, people drawn to starches first and vegetables last. *JAMA Internal Medicine, 172*(12), 961–963. doi:10.1001/archinternmed.2012.1278

98. Andrade, A. M., Greene, G. W., & Melanson, K. J. (2008). Eating slowly led to decreases in energy intake within meals in healthy women. *Journal of the American Dietetic Association, 108*(7), 1186–1191. doi:10.1016/j.jada.2008.04.026

99. Research examines vicious cycle of overeating and obesity. (2010, September 30). *ScienceDaily*. Retrieved from http://www.sciencedaily.com /releases/2010/09/100929171819.htm

100. Stice, E., Yokum, S., Blum, K., & Bohon, C. (2010). Weight gain is associated with reduced striatal response to palatable food. *Journal of Neuroscience, 30*(39), 13105–13109. doi:10.1523/JNEUROSCI.2105-10.2010

101. Speed of eating "key to obesity." (2008, October 22). *BBC News*. Retrieved from http://news.bbc.co.uk/2/hi/7681458.stm

102. Maruyama, K., Sato, S., Ohira, T., Maeda, K., Noda, H., Kubota, Y., Nishimura, S., Kitamura, A., Kiyama, M., Okada, T., Imano, H., Nakamura, M., Ishikawa, Y., Kurokawa, M., Satoshi, S., & Iso, H. (2008). The joint impact on being overweight of self reported behaviours of eating quickly and eating until full : Cross sectional survey. *British Medical Journal, 337*, a2002–a2002. doi:10.1136/bmj.a2002

103. Otsuka, R., Tamakoshi, K., Yatsuya, H., Murata, C., Sekiya, A., Wada, K., Zhang, H. M., et al. (2006). Eating fast leads to obesity: Findings based on self-administered questionnaires among middle-aged Japanese men and women. *Journal of Epidemiology, 16*(3), 117–124.

104. Eating fast increases diabetes risk. (2012, May 7). *ScienceDaily*. Retrieved from http://www.sciencedaily.com /releases/2012/05/120507210038.htm

105. Why eating too quickly is a fast track to an early grave. (2011, November 21). *Mail Online*. Retrieved from http://www.dailymail.co.uk/health/article-2064544/Why-eating-quickly-fast-track-early-grave.html

106. Sibold, J. S., & Berg, K. M. (2010). Mood enhancement persists for up to 12 hours following aerobic exercise: A pilot study. *Perceptual and Motor Skills, 111*(2), 333–342.

107. Doheny, K. (2009, May 29). Post-exercise "glow" may last 12 Hours. *US News and World Report*. Retrieved from http://health.usnews.com/health-news/family-health /brain-and-behavior/articles/2009/05/29/post-exercise-glow-may-last-12 -hours

108. Van Proeyen, K., Szlufcik, K., Nielens, H., Pelgrim, K., Deldicque, L., Hesselink, M., Van Veldhoven, P. P., & Hespel, P. (2010). Training in the fasted state improves glucose tolerance during fat-rich diet. *Journal of Physiology, 588*(21), 4289–4302. doi:10.1113/ jphysiol.2010.196493

109. Reynolds, G. (2011, September 28). How exercise can strengthen the brain. *New York Times: Well.* [Web log]. Retrieved from http://well.blogs.nytimes.com/2011/09/28/ how-exercise-can-strengthen-the-brain/

Chapter Nine

110. De Castro, J. M. (1994). Family and friends produce greater social facilitation of food intake than other companions. *Physiology & Behavior, 56*(3), 445–455. doi:10.1016/0031-9384(94)90286-0

111. De Castro, J. M. (2000). Eating behavior: Lessons from the real world of humans. *Nutrition, 16*(10), 800–13.

112. Thaler, R. H., & Sunstein, C. R. (2008). *Nudge: Improving decisions about health, wealth, and happiness.* New Haven, CT: Yale University Press.

113. Campbell, M. C., & Mohr, G. S. (2011). Seeing is eating: How and when activation of a negative stereotype increases stereotype-conducive behavior. *Journal of Consumer Research, 38*(3), 431–444.

114. Harmon, K. (2011, May 05). How obesity spreads in social networks. Retrieved from http://www.scientificamerican.com/article.cfm?id=social-spread-obesity

115. Corenman, D. (2013, January 16). Lifting techniques. Retrieved from http://neckand-back.com/pre-and-post-op/lifting-techniques

116. Bonner, F. J., Sinaki, M., Grabois, M., Shipp, K. M., Lane, J. M., Lindsay, R., Gold, D. T., Cosman, F., Bouxsein, M. L., Weinstein, J. N., Gallagher, R. M., Melton, L. J., Salcido, R. S., & Gordon, S. L. (2003). Health professional's guide to rehabilitation of the patient with osteoporosis. *Osteoporosis International, 14*(Supplement 2), S1–22. doi:10.1007/ s00198-003-1467-3

117. Chellappa, S. L., Steiner, R., Blattner, P., Oelhafen, P., Götz, T., & Cajochen, C. (2011). Non-visual effects of light on melatonin, alertness and cognitive performance: Can blue-enriched light keep us alert? *PLoS ONE, 6*(1), e16429. doi:10.1371/journal. pone.0016429

118. Gooley, J. J., Chamberlain, K., Smith, K. A., Khalsa, S. B. S., Rajaratnam, S. M. W., Van Reen, E., Zeitzer, J. M., Czeisler, C. A., & Lockley, S. W. (2011). Exposure to room light before bedtime suppresses melatonin onset and shortens melatonin duration in humans. *Journal of Clinical Endocrinology and Metabolism, 96*(3), E463–E472. doi:10.1210/ jc.2010-2098

119. Falchi, F., Cinzano, P., Elvidge, C. D., Keith, D. M., & Haim, A. (2011). Limiting the impact of light pollution on human health, environment and stellar visibility. *Journal of Environmental Management, 92*(10), 2714–2722. doi:10.1016/j. jenvman.2011.06.029

Chapter Ten

120. Karnani, M. M., Apergis-Schoute, J., Adamantidis, A., Jensen, L. T., de Lecea, L., Fugger, L., & Burdakov, D. (2011). Activation of central orexin/hypocretin neurons by dietary amino acids. *Neuron, 72*(4), 616–629. doi:10.1016/j.neuron.2011.08.027

121. Bernstein, A. M., Sun, Q., Hu, F. B., Stampfer, M. J., Manson, J. E., & Willett, W. C. (2010). Major dietary protein sources and risk of coronary heart disease in women. *Circulation, 122*(9), 876–883. doi:10.1161/CIRCULATIONAHA.109.915165

122. Goodstine, S. L., Zheng, T., Holford, T. R., Ward, B. A., Carter, D., Owens, P. H., & Mayne, S. T. (2003). Dietary (n-3)/(n-6) fatty acid ratio: Possible relationship to premenopausal but not postmenopausal breast cancer risk in U.S. women. *Journal of Nutrition, 133*(5), 1409–1414.

123. Norrish, A. E., Skeaff, C. M., Arribas, G. L., Sharpe, S. J., & Jackson, R. T. (1999). Prostate cancer risk and consumption of fish oils: A dietary biomarker-based case-control study. *British Journal of Cancer, 81*(7). doi:10.1038/sj.bjc.6690835

124. Low levels of omega-3 fatty acids may cause memory problems. (2012, February 27). *ScienceDaily*. Retrieved from http://www.sciencedaily.com / releases/2012/02/120227162549.htm

125. Swenor, B. K., Bressler, S., Caulfield, L., & West, S. K. (2010). The impact of fish and shellfish consumption on age-related macular degeneration. *Ophthalmology, 117*(12), 2395–2401. doi:10.1016/j.ophtha.2010.03.058

126. Zhao, Y.-T., Chen, Q., Sun, Y.-X., Li, X.-B., Zhang, P., Xu, Y., & Guo, J.-H. (2009). Prevention of sudden cardiac death with omega-3 fatty acids in patients with coronary heart disease: A meta-analysis of randomized controlled trials. *Annals of Medicine, 41*(4), 301–310. doi:10.1080/07853890802698834

127. Conklin, S. M., Manuck, S. B., Yao, J. K., Flory, J. D., Hibbeln, J. R., & Muldoon, M. F. (2007). High Ω-6 and low Ω-3 fatty acids are associated with depressive symptoms and neuroticism. *Psychosomatic Medicine, 69*(9), 932–934. doi:10.1097/PSY.0b013e31815aaa42

128. Tan, Z. S., Harris, W. S., Beiser, A. S., Au, R., Himali, J. J., Debette, S., Pikula, A., DeCarli, C., Wolf, P. A., Vasan, R. S., Robins, S. J., & Seshadri, S. (2012). Red blood cell omega-3 fatty acid levels and markers of accelerated brain aging. *Neurology, 78*(9), 658–664. doi:10.1212/WNL.0b013e318249f6a9

129. Kris-Etherton, P. M., Harris, W. S., & Appel, L. J. (2002). Fish consumption, fish oil, omega-3 fatty acids, and cardiovascular disease. *Circulation, 106*(21), 2747–2757. doi:10.1161/01.CIR.0000038493.65177.94

130. Wilder, D. (2011, October). Slash your risk for premature death with omega-3s. *Life Extension Magazine*. Retrieved June 1, 2013, from http://www.lef.org/magazine/mag2011/oct2011_Slash-Your-Risk-for-Premature-Death-with-Omega-3s_01.htm

131. Macchia, A., Monte, S., Pellegrini, F., Romero, M., Ferrante, D., Doval, H., D'Ettorre, A., Maggioni, A. P., & Tognoni, G. (2008). Omega-3 fatty acid supplementation reduces one-year risk of atrial fibrillation in patients hospitalized with myocardial infarction. *European Journal of Clinical Pharmacology, 64*(6), 627–634. doi:10.1007/s00228-008-0464-z

132. Laran, J. (2010). Goal management in sequential choices: Consumer choices for others are more indulgent than personal choices. *Journal of Consumer Research, 37*(2), 304–314.

133. Alford, L. (2010). What men should know about the impact of physical activity on their health. *International Journal of Clinical Practice, 64*(13), 1731–1734. doi:10.1111/j.1742-1241.2010.02478.x

134. Lifestyle could reduce cancer two-thirds. (2009, November, 16). *UPI*. Retrieved from http://www.upi.com/Health_News/2009/11/16/Lifestyle-could-reduce-cancer-two-thirds/UPI-82711258392618/

135. Eheman, C., Henley, S. J., Ballard–Barbash, R., Jacobs, E. J., Schymura, M. J., Noone, A., Pan, L., Anderson, R. N., Fulton, J. E., Kohler, B. A., Jemal, A., Ward, E., Plescia, M., Ries, L. A., & Edwards, B. K. (2012). Annual Report to the Nation on the status of cancer, 1975–2008, featuring cancers associated with excess weight and lack of sufficient physical activity. *Cancer, 118*(9), 2338–2366. doi:10.1002/cncr.27514

136. Ruden, E., Reardon, D. A., Coan, A. D., Herndon, J. E., Hornsby, W. E., West, M., Fels, D. R., Desjardins, A., Vredenburgh, J. J., Waner, E., Friedman, H., Friedman, H.

S., Peters, K. B., & Jones, L. W. (2011). Exercise behavior, functional capacity, and survival in adults with malignant recurrent glioma. *Journal of Clinical Oncology, 29*(21), 2918–2923. doi:10.1200/JCO.2011.34.9852

137. Fischetti, M. (2013, January 1). How to gain or lose 30 minutes of life every day. *Scientific American.* Retrieved from http://www.scientificamerican.com/article. cfm?id=how-to-gain-or-lose-30-minutes-of-life-everyday

138. Alford, L. (2010). What men should know about the impact of physical activity on their health. *International Journal of Clinical Practice, 64*(13), 1731–1734. doi:10.1111/j.1742-1241.2010.02478.x

Chapter Eleven

139. Paffenbarger, R. S., Gima, A. S., Laughlin, E., & Black, R. A. (1971). Characteristics of longshoremen related fatal coronary heart disease and stroke. *American Journal of Public Health, 61*(7), 1362–1370.

140. Church, T. S., Thomas, D. M., Tudor-Locke, C., Katzmarzyk, P. T., Earnest, C. P., Rodarte, R. Q., Martin, C. K., Blair, S. N., & Bouchard, C. (2011). Trends over 5 decades in U.S. occupation-related physical activity and their associations with obesity. *PLoS ONE, 6*(5), e19657. doi:10.1371/journal.pone.0019657

141. Ng, S. W., & Popkin, B. M. (2012). Time use and physical activity: A shift away from movement across the globe. *Obesity Reviews, 13*(8), 659-680. doi:10.1111/j.1467-789X.2011.00982.x

142. Brownson, R. C., Boehmer, T. K., & Luke, D. A. (2005). Declining rates of physical activity in the United States: What are the contributors? *Annual Review of Public Health, 26*(1), 421–443. doi:10.1146/annurev.publhealth.26.021304.144437

143. von Thiele Schwarz, U. & Hasson, H. (2011). Employee self-rated productivity and objective organizational production levels. *Journal of Occupational and Environmental Medicine, 53*(8), 838–844. doi:10.1097/JOM.0b013e31822589c2

144. Kosteas, V. (2012). The effect of exercise on earnings: Evidence from the NLSY. *Journal of Labor Research, 33*(2), 225–250. doi:10.1007/s12122-011-9129-2

145. Schlender, B. (n.d.). The lost Steve Jobs tapes. Retrieved April 25, 2012, from http://www.fastcompany.com/node/1826869/

146. Parker-Pope, T. (2011, May 25). Less active at work, Americans have packed on pounds. *New York Times: Well.* [Web log]. Retrieved from http://well.blogs.nytimes.com/2011/05/25/less-active-at-work-americans-have-packed-on-pounds/

147. Muhammad, L. (2012, April 13). More workers work through lunch or eat at their desks. *USA Today: Money.* Retrieved from http://www.usatoday.com/money/workplace/story/2012-04-15/lunch-at-work/54167808/1

148. Schwartz, T. (2012, June 18). Share this with your CEO. *Harvard Business Review Network Blog.* [Web log]. Retrieved from http://blogs.hbr.org/schwartz/2012/06/share-this-with-your-ceo.html

149. Kessler, R. C., Berglund, P. A., Coulouvrat, C., Hajak, G., Roth, T., Shahly, V., Shillington, A. C., Stephenson, J. J., & Walsh, J. K. (2011). Insomnia and the performance of US workers: Results from the America Insomnia Survey. *Sleep, 34*(9), 1161–1171. doi:10.5665/SLEEP.1230

150. High cost of insomnia may be a wake-up call. (2011, September 1). *USA Today.* Retrieved from http://yourlife.usatoday.com/health/story/2011-09-01/High-cost-of-insomnia-may-be-a-wake-up-call/50220690/1

151. Advocates for Auto and Highway Safety. (n.d). Truck driver fatigue. [Fact sheet]. Retrieved June 5, 2013 from http://www.saferoads.org/~saferoad/truck-driver-fatigue

152. Sleepy drivers as dangerous as drunk ones. (2012, May 31). Foxnews.com. Retrieved from http://www.foxnews.com/health/2012/05/31/study-sleepy-drivers-equally-as-dangerous-as-drunken-drivers/

153. Caldwell, J. A. (2012). Crew schedules, sleep deprivation, and aviation performance. *Current Directions in Psychological Science, 21*(2), 85–89. doi:10.1177/0963721411435842

154. Golden, F. (2010, November 17). Sleepy pilot blamed for deadly Air India crash. *AOL Travel News.* Retrieved from http://news.travel.aol.com/2010/11/17/sleepy-pilot-blamed-for-deadly-air-india-crash/

155. The better off sleep better. (2011, March 4). *ScienceDaily.* Retrieved from http://www.sciencedaily.com /releases/2011/03/110304091500.htm

Chapter Twelve

156. Shellenbarger, S. (2012, March 15). Colleagues who can make you fat. (2012, March 15). *Wall Street Journal.* Retrieved from http://online.wsj.com/article/SB10001424052702303717304577279402522090464.html

157. Heaner, M. (2004, October 12). Snooze alarm takes its toll on a nation. *The New York Times.* Retrieved from http://www.nytimes.com/2004/10/12/health/12snoo.html

Chapter Thirteen

158. Dr. William Davis's Wheat-Loss Diet. (n.d.) *The 700 Club.* Retrieved June 5, 2013 from http://www.cbn.com/700club/guests/bios/william_davis_101711.aspx

159. Davis, W. (2011). *Wheat belly: Lose the wheat, lose the weight, and find your path back to health.* New York: Rodale Books.

160. Jenkins, D. J., Wolever, T. M., Taylor, R. H., Barker, H., Fielden, H., Baldwin, J. M., Bowling, A. C., Newman, H. C., Jenkins, A. L., & Goff, D. V. (1981). Glycemic Index of foods: A physiological basis for carbohydrate exchange. *American Journal of Clinical Nutrition, 34*(3), 362–366.

161. Foods identified as "whole grain" not always healthy. (2013, January 10). *ScienceDaily.* Retrieved from http://www.sciencedaily.com/releases/2013/01/130110170827.htm

162. Davis, W. (2011). *Wheat belly: Lose the wheat, lose the weight, and find your path back to health.* New York: Rodale Books.

163. Collier, B., Dossett, L. A., May, A. K., & Diaz, J. J. (2008). Glucose control and the inflammatory response. *Nutrition in Clinical Practice, 23*(1), 3–15. doi:10.1177/011542650802300103

164. Stix, G. (2008, November 9). Is chronic inflammation the key to unlocking the mysteries of cancer?: *Scientific American.* Retrieved from http://www.scientificamerican.com/article.cfm?id=chronic-inflammation-cancer

165. Moyer, M. W. (2010, April 27). Carbs against cardio: More evidence that refined carbohydrates, not fats, threaten the heart: *Scientific American.* Retrieved from http://www.scientificamerican.com/article.cfm?id=carbs-against-cardio&page=2

166. University of Chicago Press Journals (2012, May 16). You are what you eat: Why do male consumers avoid vegetarian options? *ScienceDaily.* Retrieved from http://www.sciencedaily.com /releases/2012/05/120516152532.htm

167. Mozaffarian, D., Hao, T., Rimm, E. B., Willett, W. C., & Hu, F. B. (2011). Changes in diet and lifestyle and long-term weight gain in women and men. *New England Journal of Medicine, 364*, 2392-2404. doi:10.1056/NEJMoa1014296

168. Larsson, S. C., & Wolk, A. (2012). Red and processed meat consumption and risk of pancreatic cancer: Meta-analysis of prospective studies. *British Journal of Cancer, 106*(3), 603–607. doi:10.1038/bjc.2011.585

169. Pan, A., Sun, Q., Bernstein, A. M., Schulze, M. B., Manson, J. E., Willett, W. C., & Hu, F. B. (2011). Red meat consumption and risk of type 2 diabetes: 3 cohorts of US adults and an updated meta-analysis. *American Journal of Clinical Nutrition, 94*(4), 1088-1096. doi:10.3945/ajcn.111.018978

170. Bakalar, N. (2012, March 12). Red meat linked to cancer and heart disease. *The New York Times.* Retrieved from http://www.nytimes.com/2012/03/13/health/research/red-meat-linked-to-cancer-and-heart-disease.html

171. Pan, A., Sun, Q., Bernstein, A. M., Schulze, M. B., Manson, J. E., Stampfer, M. J., Willett, W. C., & Hu, F. B. (2012). Red meat consumption and mortality: Results from 2 prospective cohort studies. *Archives of Internal Medicine, 172*(7), 555–563. doi:10.1001/archinternmed.2011.2287

172. Kaluza, J., Wolk, A., & Larsson, S. C. (2012). Red meat consumption and risk of stroke a meta-analysis of prospective studies. *Stroke, 43*(10), 2556-2560. doi:10.1161/STROKEAHA.112.663286

173. Doheny, K. (2010, March 29). Can't sleep? Adjust the temperature. *WebMD*. Retrieved from http://www.webmd.com/sleep-disorders/features/cant-sleep-adjust-the-temperature

174. Kloc, J. (2011, December 21). Putting insomnia on ice. *Scientific American*. Retrieved from http://www.scientificamerican.com/article.cfm?id=putting-insomnia-on-ice

175. Beckford, M. (2011, June 13). Keep a cool head to avoid sleeplessness. *The Telegraph*. Retrieved from http://www.telegraph.co.uk/health/healthnews/8568966/Keep-a-cool-head-to-avoid-sleeplessness.html

176. Johnson, F., Mavrogianni, A., Ucci, M., Vidal–Puig, A., & Wardle, J. (2011). Could increased time spent in a thermal comfort zone contribute to population increases in obesity? *Obesity Reviews, 12*(7), 543–551. doi:10.1111/j.1467-789X.2010.00851.x.

Chapter Fourteen

177. Wansink, B., Painter, J. E., & North, J. (2005). Bottomless bowls: Why visual cues of portion size may influence intake. *Obesity, 13*(1), 93–100. doi:10.1038/oby.2005.12

178. Rolls, B. J., Morris, E. L., & Roe, L. S. (2002). Portion size of food affects energy intake in normal-weight and overweight men and women. *American Journal of Clinical Nutrition, 76*(6), 1207–1213.

179. Mindless eating: Losing weight without thinking. (2011, August 6). *ScienceDaily*. Retrieved from http://www.sciencedaily.com /releases/2011/08/110805163541.htm

180. Van Ittersum, K., & Wansink, B. (2012). Plate size and color suggestibility: The Delboeuf Illusion's bias on serving and eating behavior. *Journal of Consumer Research, 39*(2), 215 – 228.

181. Thomas, J. G., Bond, D. S., Hill, J. O., & Wing, R. R. (2011). The National Weight Control Registry (NWCR): A study of "Successful Losers." *American College of Sports Medicine Health & Fitness Journal, 15*(2).8-12. doi:10.1249/FIT.0b013e31820b72b5

182. Gruber, R., Cassoff, J., Frenette, S., Wiebe, S., & Carrier, J. (2012). Impact of sleep extension and restriction on children's emotional ability and impulsivity. *Pediatrics, 130*(5), e1155–e1161. doi:10.1542/peds.2012-0564

183. Mindell, J. A., Meltzer, L. J., Carskadon, M. A., & Chervin, R. D. (2009). Developmental aspects of sleep hygiene: Findings from the 2004 National Sleep Foundation Sleep in America Poll. *Sleep Medicine, 10*(7), 771–779. doi:10.1016/j.sleep.2008.07.016

184. Stone, M. R., Stevens, D., & Faulkner, G. E. J. (2013). Maintaining recommended sleep throughout the week is associated with increased physical activity in children. *Preventive Medicine, 56*(2), 112–117. doi:10.1016/j.ypmed.2012.11.015

185. Golley, R. K., Maher, C. A., Matricciani, L., & Olds, T. S. (2013). Sleep duration or bedtime? Exploring the association between sleep timing behaviour, diet and BMI in children and adolescents. *International Journal of Obesity, 37*(4), 546-551. doi:10.1038/ijo.2012.212

Chapter Fifteen

186. Wilcox, K., Vallen, B., Block, L., & Fitzsimons, G. J. (2009). Vicarious goal fulfillment: When the mere presence of a healthy option leads to an ironically indulgent decision. *Journal of Consumer Research, 36*(3), 380–393. doi: 10.1086/599219

187. Wu, H. W. & Sturm, R. (2012). What's on the menu? A review of the energy and nutritional content of US chain restaurant menus. *Public Health Nutrition, 16*(1), 87-96. doi:10.1017/S136898001200122X

188. Ruby, M. B., Dunn, E. W., Perrino, A., Gillis, R., & Viel, S. (2011). The invisible benefits of exercise. *Health Psychology, 30*(1), 67–74. doi:10.1037/a0021859

189. Redelmeier, D. A., & Kahneman, D. (1996). Patients' memories of painful medical treatments: Real-time and retrospective evaluations of two minimally invasive procedures. *Pain, 66*(1), 3–8. doi:10.1016/0304-3959(96)02994-6

190. Gilovich, T., Griffin, D. W., & Kahneman, D. (2002). *Heuristics and biases: The psychology of intuitive judgment.* New York: Cambridge University Press.

191. O'Brien, E., & Ellsworth, P. C. (2012). Saving the last for best: A positivity bias for end experiences. *Psychological Science, 23*(2), 163-165. doi:10.1177/0956797611427408

192. Weiser, P. (2010, June 21) Cool down and enjoy. *Endurance Education.* Retrieved from http://www.endurance-education.com/pushing-the-envelope/cool-down-and-enjoy/

193. SoundaraPandian, S., Ekkekakis, P., & Welch, A. S. (2010). Exercise as an affective experience: Does adding a positive end impact future exercise choice? *Medicine & Science in Sports & Exercise, 42*(5), 102–103. doi:10.1249/01.MSS.0000385962.64835.7a

194. Kolata, G. (2012, November 19). Updating the message to get Americans moving. *New York Times: Well.* [Web log]. Retrieved January 17, 2013, from http://well.blogs.nytimes.com/2012/11/19/updating-the-message-to-get-americans-moving/

195. Fenn, K. M., & Hambrick, D. Z. (2011). Individual differences in working memory capacity predict sleep-dependent memory consolidation. *Journal of Experimental Psychology: General, 141*(3), 404-410. doi:10.1037/a0025268

196. Wilhelm, I., Diekelmann, S., Molzow, I., Ayoub, A., Mölle, M., & Born, J. (2011). Sleep selectively enhances memory expected to be of future relevance. *Journal of Neuroscience, 31*(5), 1563–1569. doi:10.1523/JNEUROSCI.3575-10.2011

197. Ferrie, J. E., Shipley, M. J., Akbaraly, T. N., Marmot, M. G., Kivimäki, M., & Singh-Manoux, A. (2011). Change in sleep duration and cognitive function: Findings from the Whitehall II Study. *Sleep, 34*(5), 565–573.

Chapter Sixteen

198. Diet linked to daytime sleepiness and alertness in healthy adults. (2013, May 7). *ScienceDaily.* Retrieved from http://www.sciencedaily.com /releases/2013/05/130507164632.htm

199. Golomb, B. A., Evans, M. A., White, H. L., & Dimsdale, J. E. (2012). Trans fat consumption and aggression. *PLoS ONE, 7*(3), e32175. doi:10.1371/journal.pone.0032175

200. More trans fat consumption linked to greater aggression, researchers find. (2012, March 13). *ScienceDaily.* Retrieved from http://www.sciencedaily.com / releases/2012/03/120313122504.htm

201. Sánchez-Villegas, A., Toledo, E., de Irala, J., Ruiz-Canela, M., Pla-Vidal, J., & Martínez-González, M. A. (2012). Fast-food and commercial baked goods consumption and the risk of depression. *Public Health Nutrition, 15*(3), 424–432. doi:10.1017/S1368980011001856

202. High-fat diet may make you stupid and lazy. (n.d.). *LiveScience.com.* Retrieved June 6, 2013, from http://www.livescience.com/5635-high-fat-diet-stupid-lazy.html

203. Does fatty food impact marital stress? (2012, April 24). *ScienceDaily.* Retrieved from http://www.sciencedaily.com/releases/2012/04/120424095502.htm

204. Many apples a day keep the blues at bay. (2013, January 23). *ScienceDaily.* Retrieved from http://www.sciencedaily.com /releases/2013/01/130123195351.htm

205. Griffin, É. W., Mullally, S., Foley, C., Warmington, S. A., O'Mara, S. M., & Kelly, Á. M. (2011). Aerobic exercise improves hippocampal function and increases BDNF in

the serum of young adult males. *Physiology & Behavior, 104*(5), 934–941. doi:10.1016/j. physbeh.2011.06.005

206. Walking slows progression of Alhzeimer's, study shows. (2010, November 29). *Science-Daily*. Retrieved from http://www.sciencedaily.com /releases/2010/11/101129101914. htm

207. Woodcock, J., Franco, O. H., Orsini, N., & Roberts, I. (2011). Non-vigorous physical activity and all-cause mortality: Systematic review and meta-analysis of cohort studies. *International Journal of Epidemiology, 40*(1), 121-138 doi:10.1093/ije/dyq104

208. Loprinzi, P. D., & Cardinal, B. J. (2011). Association between objectively-measured physical activity and sleep, NHANES 2005–2006. *Mental Health and Physical Activity, 4*(2), 65–69. doi:10.1016/j.mhpa.2011.08.001

209. Physical activity impacts overall quality of sleep. (2011, November 22). *ScienceDaily*. Retrieved from http://www.sciencedaily.com /releases/2011/11/111122143354.htm

210. Exercising close to bedtime is OK, sleep experts say. (2013, March 4). *USA Today*. Retrieved from http://www.usatoday.com/story/news/nation/2013/03/04/ sleep-survey-exercise-insomnia/1955117/

Chapter Seventeen

211. Hofmann, W., Baumeister, R. F., Förster, G., & Vohs, K. D. (2011). Everyday temptations: An experience sampling study of desire, conflict, and self-control. *Journal of Personality and Social Psychology, 102*(6), 1318-1335. doi:10.1037/a0026545

212. Allen, G. J., & Albala, K. (2007). *The business of food: Encyclopedia of the food and drink industries*. Westport, CT: ABC-CLIO.

213. Schuldt, J. P., Muller, D., & Schwarz, N. (2012). The "Fair Trade" effect: Health halos from social ethics claims. *Social Psychological and Personality Science*. doi:10.1177/1948550611431643

214. Lee, W. J., Shimizu, M., Kniffin, K. M., & Wansink, B. (2013). You taste what you see: Do organic labels bias taste perceptions? *Food Quality and Preference, 29*(1), 33–39. doi:10.1016/j.foodqual.2013.01.010

215. Lloyd, J. (2011, June 13). Apples top most pesticide-contaminated list. *USA Today*. Retrieved from http://yourlife.usatoday.com/fitness-food/safety/story/2011/06/ Apples-top-list-of-produce-contaminated-with-pesticides/48332000/1

216. Gokee LaRose, J. Leahey, T. M., Weinberg, B. M., Kumar, R., & Wing, R. R. (2012). Young adults' performance in a low-Intensity weight loss campaign. *Obesity, 20*(11), 2314-2316. doi:10.1038/oby.2012.30

217. Bault, N., Joffily, M., Rustichini, A., & Coricelli, G. (2011). Medial prefrontal cortex and striatum mediate the influence of social comparison on the decision process. *Proceedings of the National Academy of Sciences, 108*(38), 16044-16049. doi:10.1073/ pnas.1100892108

Chapter Eighteen

218. Smith, K. J., Gall, S. L., McNaughton, S. A., Blizzard, L., Dwyer, T., & Venn, A. J. (2010). Skipping breakfast: Longitudinal associations with cardiometabolic risk factors in the Childhood Determinants of Adult Health Study. *American Journal of Clinical Nutrition, 92*(6), 1316–1325. doi:10.3945/ajcn.2010.30101

219. Clendaniel, M. (n.d.). People who eat breakfast are smarter and skinnier. *Co.Exist*. Retrieved July 1, 2013 from http://www.fastcoexist.com/1680410/people-who-eat-breakfast-are-smarter-and-skinnier

220. Kiefer, I. (2007). Brain food. *Scientific American Mind, 18*(5), 58–63. doi:10.1038/ scientificamericanmind1007-58

221. Glycemic index foods at breakfast can control blood sugar throughout the day. (2012, March 30). *ScienceDaily*. Retrieved from http://www.sciencedaily.com/releases/ 2012/03/120330110204.htm

222. Leidy, H. J., Ortinau, L. C., Douglas, S. M., & Hoertel, H. A. (2013). Beneficial effects of a higher-protein breakfast on the appetitive, hormonal, and neural signals controlling energy intake regulation in overweight/obese, "breakfast-skipping," late-adolescent girls. *American Journal of Clinical Nutrition, 97*(4), 677–688. doi:10.3945/ajcn.112.053116

223. Wilson, M. (n.d.). Infographic: When the lights go out, the world eats junk. *Co.Design.* Retrieved July 1, 2013 from http://www.fastcodesign.com/1669761/infographic-when-the-lights-go-out-the-world-eats-junk

224. St-Onge, M. P., McReynolds, A., Trivedi, Z. B., Roberts, A. L., Sy, M., & Hirsch, J. (2012). Sleep restriction leads to increased activation of brain regions sensitive to food stimuli. *American Journal of Clinical Nutrition, 95*(4), 818-824. doi:10.3945/ajcn.111.027383

225. Stamatakis, E., Hamer, M., & Dunstan, D. W. (2011). Screen-based entertainment time, all-cause mortality, and cardiovascular events: Population-based study with ongoing mortality and hospital events follow-up. *Journal of the American College of Cardiology, 57*(3), 292–299. doi:10.1016/j.jacc.2010.05.065

226. Veerman, J. L., Healy, G. N., Cobiac, L. J., Vos, T., Winkler, E. A. H., Owen, N., & Dunstan, D. W. (2011). Television viewing time and reduced life expectancy: A life table analysis. *British Journal of Sports Medicine, 46*(13), 927-930. doi:10.1136/bjsm.2011.085662

227. Shaw, M. (2000). Time for a smoke? One cigarette reduces your life by 11 minutes. *BMJ, 320*(7226), 53–53. doi:10.1136/bmj.320.7226.53

228. Get up. Get out. Don't sit. (2012, October 17). *New York Times: Well.* [Web log]. Retrieved from http://well.blogs.nytimes.com/2012/10/17/get-up-get-out-dont-sit/

229. Veerman, J. L., Healy, G. N., Cobiac, L. J., Vos, T., Winkler, E. A. H., Owen, N., & Dunstan, D. W. (2011). Television viewing time and reduced life expectancy: A life table analysis. *British Journal of Sports Medicine, 46*(13), 927-930. doi:10.1136/bjsm.2011.085662

230. Steeves, J. A., Thompson, D. L., & Bassett, D. R. (2012). Energy cost of stepping in place while watching television commercials. *Medicine & Science in Sports & Exercise, 44*(2), 330–335. doi:10.1249/MSS.0b013e31822d797e

231. Sleepy connected Americans. (2011, March 7). *ScienceDaily.* Retrieved from http://www.sciencedaily.com /releases/2011/03/110307065350.htm

232. O'Connor, A. (2012, September 10). Really? Using a computer before bed can disrupt sleep. *New York Times: Well.* [Web log]. Retrieved from http://well.blogs.nytimes.com/2012/09/10/really-using-a-computer-before-bed-can-disrupt-sleep/

233. Wood, B., Rea, M. S., Plitnick, B., & Figueiro, M. G. (2012). Light level and duration of exposure determine the impact of self-luminous tablets on melatonin suppression. *Applied Ergonomics, 44*(2), 237-240. doi:10.1016/j.apergo.2012.07.008

Chapter Nineteen

234. USDA National Nutrient Database for Standard Reference. (2013). Nutrient data for 09003, apples, raw, with skin. [Nutritional analysis]. Retrieved from http://ndb.nal.usda.gov/ndb/foods/show/2141?fg=&man=&lfacet=&format=&count=&max=25&offset=&sort=&qlookup=apple

235. USDA National Nutrient Database for Standard Reference. (2013). Nutrient data for 09400, apple juice, canned or bottled, unsweetened, with added ascorbic acid. [Nutritional analysis]. Retrieved from http://ndb.nal.usda.gov/ndb/foods/show/2423?fg=&man=&lfacet=&format=&count=&max=25&offset=&sort=&qlookup=apple+juice

236. Harvard School of Public Health. (2012). *How sweet is it? Calories and teaspoons of sugar in 12 ounces of each beverage.* [Graph illustration]. Retrieved from http://www.hsph.harvard.edu/nutritionsource/files/2012/10/how-sweet-is-it-color.pdf

237. Hold the diet soda? Sweetened drinks linked to depression, coffee tied to lower risk. (2013, January 8). *ScienceDaily.* Retrieved from http://www.sciencedaily.com/releases/2013/01/130108162135.htm

238. Fat Secret. (2013). 1 cup dried mango. [Nutritional analysis]. Retrieved from http://www.fatsecret.com/calories-nutrition/generic/mango-dried?portionid=22479&portionamount=1.000

239. USDA National Nutrient Database for Standard Reference. (2013). Nutrient data for19110, candies, Krackel chocolate bar. [Nutritional analysis]. Retrieved from http://ndb.nal.usda.gov/ndb/foods/show/5914?fg=&man=&lfacet=&format=&count=&max=25&offset=0&sort=&qlookup=candy+bar

240. Ipatenco, S. (n.d.). Are dried cranberries good for you? *San Francisco Chronicle: Healthy Eating.* Retrieved March 19, 2013, from http://healthyeating.sfgate.com/dried-cranberries-good-you-3668.html

241. Irmak, C., Vallen, B., & Robinson, S. R. (2011). The impact of product name on dieters' and nondieters' food evaluations and consumption. *Journal of Consumer Research, 38*(2), 390–405.

242. Froot Loops Doctor Commercial [Video file]. Retrieved June 6, 2013 from http://www.youtube.com/watch?v=Br3gdKguUx0&feature=youtube_gdata_player

243. Kellogg's® Froot Loops® cereal. (n.d.). Retrieved June 6, 2013 from from http://www2.kelloggs.com/ProductDetail.aspx?id=566

244. My Fitness Pal. (2013). *Calories in egg white omelette with bell pepper tomato and veggie sausage.* [Computation of nutritional content]. Retrieved from http://www.myfitnesspal.com/food/calories/egg-white-omelette-egg-white-omelette-with-bell-pepper-tomato-and-veggie-sausage-8100420

245. Mandal, B. (2010). Use of food labels as a weight loss behavior. *Journal of Consumer Affairs, 44*(3), 516–527, 527. doi:10.1111/j.1745-6606.2010.01181.x

246. Schuldt, J. P. (2013). Does green mean healthy? Nutrition label color affects perceptions of healthfulness. *Health Communication,* 1-8. doi: 10.1080/10410236.2012.725270

247. Lapierre, M. A., Vaala, S. E., & Linebarger, D. L. (2011). Influence of licensed spokescharacters and health cues on children's ratings of cereal taste. *Archives of Pediatric and Adolescent Medicine, 165*(3), 229–234. doi:10.1001/archpediatrics.2010.300

248. Elliott, C. D. (2011). Sweet and salty: Nutritional content and analysis of baby and toddler foods. *Journal of Public Health, 33*(1), 63–70. doi:10.1093/pubmed/fdq037

249. Zhou, J., Liu, D., Li, X., Ma, J., Zhang, J., & Fang, J. (2012). Pink noise: Effect on complexity synchronization of brain activity and sleep consolidation. *Journal of Theoretical Biology, 306,* 68–72. doi:10.1016/j.jtbi.2012.04.006

Chapter Twenty

250. Charred meat may increase risk of pancreatic cancer. (2009, April 21). *ScienceDaily.* Retrieved from http://www.sciencedaily.com /releases/2009/04/090421154327.htm

251. Cai, W., Ramdas, M., Zhu, L., Chen, X., Striker, G. E., & Vlassara, H. (2012). Oral advanced glycation endproducts (AGEs) promote insulin resistance and diabetes by depleting the antioxidant defenses AGE receptor-1 and sirtuin 1. *Proceedings of the National Academy of Sciences, 109*(39), 15888-15893. doi: 10.1073/pnas.1205847109

252. Food preparation may play a big role in chronic disease. (2007, April 24). *ScienceDaily.* Retrieved from http://www.sciencedaily.com /releases/2007/04/070424155559.htm

253. Luevano-Contreras, C., Garay-Sevilla, M. E., Preciado-Puga, M., & Chapman-Novakofski, K. M. (2013). The relationship between dietary advanced glycation end products and indicators of diabetes severity in Mexicans and non-Hispanic whites: A pilot study. *International Journal of Food Sciences and Nutrition, 64*(1), 16–20. doi:10.3109/09637486.2012.704905

254. Guillén, M. D., & Uriarte, P. S. (2012). Aldehydes contained in edible oils of a very different nature after prolonged heating at frying temperature: Presence of toxic oxygenated α,β unsaturated aldehydes. *Food Chemistry, 131*(3), 915–926. doi:10.1016/j.foodchem.2011.09.079

255. Jacobson, S. H., King, D. M., & Yuan, R. (2011). A note on the relationship between obesity and driving. *Transport Policy, 18*(5), 772–776. doi:10.1016/j.tranpol.2011.03.008

256. Reich, K. A., Chen, Y.-W., Thompson, P. D., Hoffman, E. P., & Clarkson, P. M. (2010). Forty-eight hours of unloading and 24 h of reloading lead to changes in global gene expression patterns related to ubiquitination and oxidative stress in humans. *Journal of Applied Physiology, 109*(5), 1404–1415. doi:10.1152/japplphysiol.00444.2010

257. Long commutes "bad for marriage": Swedish study. (2011, May 24). *The Local.* Retrieved from http://www.thelocal.se/33966/20110524/#.UPgHzytddiQ

258. Lowrey, A. (2011, May 26). Your commute is killing you. *Slate.* Retrieved from http://www.slate.com/articles/business/moneybox/2011/05/your_commute_is_killing_you.single.html

259. Stutzer, A., & Frey, B. S. (2008). Stress that doesn't pay: The commuting paradox. *Scandinavian Journal of Economics, 110*(2), 339-366. doi: 10.1111/j.1467-9442.2008.00542.x

260. Wang, S. S. (2011, March 29). How your schedule can help (or hurt) your health. *Wall Street Journal.* Retrieved from http://online.wsj.com/article/SB10001424052748704471904576228532850374342.html?mod=rss_Health#printMode

261. Heart attacks rise following daylight saving time. (2012, March 7). *ScienceDaily.* Retrieved from http://www.sciencedaily.com /releases/2012/03/120307162555.htm

262. Mazzoccoli, G., Piepoli, A., Carella, M., Panza, A., Pazienza, V., Benegiamo, G., Palumbo, O., & Ranieri, E. (2012). Altered expression of the clock gene machinery in kidney cancer patients. *Biomedicine & Pharmacotherapy, 66*(3), 175-179. doi:10.1016/j.biopha.2011.11.007

263. O'Connor, A. (2012, May 20). Sleep apnea tied to increased cancer risk. *New York Times: Well.* [Web log]. Retrieved from http://well.blogs.nytimes.com/2012/05/20/sleep-apnea-tied-to-increased-cancer-risk

264. Buxton, O. M., Cain, S. W., O'Connor, S. P., Porter, J. H., Duffy, J. F., Wang, W., Czeisler, C. A., & Shea, S. A. (2012). Adverse metabolic consequences in humans of prolonged sleep restriction combined with circadian disruption. *Science Translational Medicine, 4*(129), 129ra43–129ra43. doi:10.1126/scitranslmed.3003200

Chapter Twenty-One

265. Pollan, M. (2009). *Food rules: An eater's manual.* New York: Penguin.

266. How long do canned meats last? (n.d.). *Eat By Date.* Retrieved June 8, 2013 from http://www.eatbydate.com/proteins/meats/how-long-does-canned-meat-last-shelf-life-expiration-date/

267. Darrington, J. (2008). White rice. *Utah State University Cooperative Extension.* Retrieved June 8, 2013 from http://extension.usu.edu/foodstorage/htm/white-rice

268. Bohns, V. K. & Wiltermuth, S. S. (2012). It hurts when I do this (or you do that): Posture and pain tolerance. *Journal of Experimental Social Psychology, 48*(1), 341–345. doi:10.1016/j.jesp.2011.05.022

269. Briñol, P., Petty, R. E., & Wagner, B. (2009). Body posture effects on self–evaluation: A self–validation approach. *European Journal of Social Psychology, 39*(6), 1053–1064. doi:10.1002/ejsp.607

270. Alderman, L. (2011, June 24). Sit up straight to avoid back problems. *New York Times.* Retrieved from http://www.nytimes.com/2011/06/25/health/25consumer.html

271. Epstein, R. (2011, September 08). Fight the frazzled mind: Proactive steps manage stress. *Scientific American.* Retrieved from http://www.scientificamerican.com/article.cfm?id=fight-the-frazzled-mind

272. Ackermann, K., Revell, V. L., Lao, O., Rombouts, E. J., Skene, D. J., & Kayser, M. (2012). Diurnal rhythms in blood cell populations and the effect of acute sleep deprivation in healthy young men. *Sleep, 35*(7), 933-940. doi:10.5665/sleep.1954

273. Campbell, J. P., Karolak, M. R., Ma, Y., Perrien, D. S., Masood-Campbell, S. K., Penner, N. L., Munoz, S. A., Zijlstra, A., Yang, X., Sterling, J. A., & Eleftriou, F. (2012). Stimulation of host bone marrow stromal cells by sympathetic nerves promotes breast cancer bone metastasis in mice. *PLoS Biol, 10*(7), e1001363. doi:10.1371/journal.pbio.1001363

274. Piazza, J. R., Charles, S. T., Sliwinski, M. J., Almeida, D. M. (2012). Affective reactivity to daily stressors and long-term risk of reporting a chronic physical health condition. *Annals of Behavioral Medicine, 45*(1), 110–120. doi:10.1007/s12160-012-9423-0

275. Reactions to everyday stressors predict future health. (2012, November 2). *ScienceDaily.* Retrieved from http://www.sciencedaily.com /releases/2012/11/121102205143.htm

Chapter Twenty-Two

276. Stephen, I. D., Coetzee, V., & Perrett, D. I. (2011). Carotenoid and melanin pigment coloration affect perceived human health. *Evolution and Human Behavior, 32*(3), 216–227. doi:10.1016/j.evolhumbehav.2010.09.003

277. Eating vegetables gives skin a more healthy glow than the sun, study shows. (2011, January 11). *ScienceDaily.* Retrieved from http://www.sciencedaily.com / releases/2011/01/110111133224.htm

278. Krieger, E. B. (n.d.). Top 10 foods for healthy hair. *WebMD.* Retrieved March 15, 2013 from http://www.webmd.com/healthy-beauty/features/top-10-foods-for-healthy-hair

279. Skin problems and treatments. (n.d.). *WebMD.* Retrieved June 5, 2013 from http:// www.webmd.com/skin-problems-and-treatments/picture-of-the-hair

280. Krieger, E. B. (n.d.). Top 10 foods for healthy hair. *WebMD.* Retrieved March 15, 2013 from http://www.webmd.com/healthy-beauty/features/top-10-foods-for-healthy-hair

281. Safdar, A., Bourgeois, J. M., Ogborn, D. I., Little, J. P., Hettinga, B. P., Akhtar, M., Thompson, J. E., Melov, S., Mocellin, N. J., Kujoth, G. C., Prolla, T. A., & Tarnopolsky, M. A. (2011). Endurance exercise rescues progeroid aging and induces systemic mitochondrial rejuvenation in mtDNA mutator mice. *Proceedings of the National Academy of Sciences, 108*(10), 4135-4140. doi:10.1073/pnas.1019581108

282. Reynolds, G. (2011, March 2). Can exercise keep you young? *New York Times: Well.* [Web log]. Retrieved from http://well.blogs.nytimes.com/2011/03/02/can-exercise-keep-you-young/

283. Gielen, S., Sandri, M., Kozarez, I., Kratzsch, J., Teupser, D., Thiery, J., Erbs, S., Mangner, N., Lenk, K., Hambrecht, R., Schuler, G., & Adams, V. (2012). Exercise training attenuates MuRF-1 expression in the skeletal muscle of patients with chronic heart failure independent of age: The Randomized Leipzig Exercise Intervention in Chronic Heart Failure and Aging (LEICA) Catabolism Study. *Circulation, 125*(22), 2716-2727. doi:10.1161/CIRCULATIONAHA.111.047381

284. Axelsson, J., Sundelin, T., Ingre, M., Van Someren, E. J. W., Olsson, A., & Lekander, M. (2010). Beauty sleep: Experimental study on the perceived health and attractiveness of sleep deprived people. *British Medical Journal, 341*, c6614–c6614. doi: http://dx.doi.org/10.1136/bmj.c6614

285. Altemus, M., Rao, B., Dhabhar, F. S., Ding, W., & Granstein, R. D. (2001). Stress-induced changes in skin barrier function in healthy women. *Journal of Investigative Dermatology, 117*(2), 309–317. doi:10.1046/j.1523-1747.2001.01373.x

Chapter Twenty-Three

286. Wansink, B., Aner, T., & Shimzu, M. (2012). First foods most: After 18-hour fast, people drawn to starches first and vegetables last. *Archives of Internal Medicine, 172*(12), 961–963. doi:10.1001/archinternmed.2012.1278

287. O'Connor, A. (2012, June 26). Craving carbs on an empty stomach. *New York Times: Well.* [Web log] Retrieved from http://well.blogs.nytimes.com/2012/06/26/craving-carbs-on-an-empty-stomach/

288. Drink water to curb weight gain? Clinical trial confirms effectiveness of simple appetite control method. (2010, August 23). *ScienceDaily*. Retrieved from http://www.sciencedaily.com /releases/2010/08/100823142929.htm

289. Kolata, G. (2012, November 19). Updating the message to get Americans moving. *New York Times: Well*. [Web log] Retrieved from http://well.blogs.nytimes.com/2012/11/19/updating-the-message-to-get-americans-moving/

290. Exercise and addiction: Fun run. (2012, April 14).*The Economist*. Retrieved from http://www.economist.com/node/21552536

291. Raichlen, D. A., Foster, A. D., Gerdeman, G. L., Seillier, A., & Giuffrida, A. (2012). Wired to run: Exercise-induced endocannabinoid signaling in humans and cursorial mammals with implications for the "runner's high". *Journal of Experimental Biology, 215*(8), 1331–1336. doi:10.1242/jeb.063677

292. Joyce, C. (2012, May 7). 'Wired to run': Runner's high may have been evolutionary advantage. *NPR: Shots*. Retrieved from http://www.npr.org/blogs/health/2012/05/07/151936266/wired-to-run-runners-high-may-have-been-evolutionary-advantage

293. Squatriglia, C. (2012, May 3). Study reveals joggers live 5 years longer. *WIRED*. Retrieved from http://www.wired.com/playbook/2012/05/joggers-live-longer/

294. van der Helm, E., Yao, J., Dutt, S., Rao, V., Saletin, J. M., & Walker, M. P. (2011). REM sleep depotentiates amygdala activity to previous emotional experiences. *Current Biology, 21*(23), 2029–2032. doi:10.1016/j.cub.2011.10.052

295. Dreaming takes the sting out of painful memories, research shows. (2011, November 23). *ScienceDaily*. Retrieved from http://www.sciencedaily.com /releases/2011/11/111123133346.htm

296. Griffith, L. C., & Rosbash, M. (2008). Sleep: Hitting the reset button. *Nature Neuroscience, 11*(2), 123–124. doi:10.1038/nn0208-123

297. Castro, J. (2012). Sleep's secret repairs. *Scientific American Mind, 23*(2), 42–45. doi:10.1038/scientificamericanmind0512-42

Chapter Twenty-Four

298. Wiecha, J. L., Peterson, K. E., Ludwig, D. S., Kim, J., Sobol, A., & Gortmaker, S. L. (2006). When children eat what they watch: Impact of television viewing on dietary intake in youth. *Archives of Pediatric and Adolescent Medicine, 160*(4), 436–442. doi:10.1001/archpedi.160.4.436

299. Neal, D. T., Wood, W., Wu, M., & Kurlander, D. (2011). The pull of the past: When do habits persist despite conflict with motives? *Personality and Social Psychology Bulletin, 37*(11), 1428–1437. doi:10.1177/0146167211419863

300. Geier, A., Wansink, B., & Rozin, P. (2012). Red potato chips: Segmentation cues can substantially decrease food intake. *Health Psychology, 31*(3), 398–401. doi:10.1037/a0027221

301. Thompson Coon, J., Boddy, K., Stein, K., Whear, R., Barton, J., & Depledge, M. H. (2011). Does participating in physical activity in outdoor natural environments have a greater effect on physical and mental wellbeing than physical activity indoors? A systematic review. *Environmental Science and Technology, 45*(5), 1761–1772. doi:10.1021/es102947t

302. In the green of health: Just 5 minutes of 'green exercise' optimal for good mental health. (2010, May 21). *ScienceDaily*. Retrieved from http://www.sciencedaily.com /releases/2010/05/100502080414.htm

303. Helliker, K. (2010, May 18). The power of a gentle nudge: Phone calls, even voice recordings, can get people to go to the gym. *Wall Street Journal*. Retrieved from http://online.wsj.com/article/SB10001424052748704314904575250352409843386.html

304. King, A. C., Friedman, R., Marcus, B., Castro, C., Napolitano, M., Ahn, D., & Baker, L. (2007). Ongoing physical activity advice by humans versus computers: The

Community Health Advice by Telephone (CHAT) trial. *Health Psychology, 26*(6), 718–727. doi:10.1037/0278-6133.26.6.718

305. Helliker, K. (2010, May 18). The power of a gentle nudge: Phone calls, even voice recordings, can get people to go to the gym. *Wall Street Journal.* Retrieved from http://online.wsj.com/article/SB10001424052748704314904575250352409843386.html

306. Optimal workout partner encourages less to motivate more. (2013, May 7) *ScienceDaily.* Retrieved from http://www.sciencedaily.com/releases/2013/05/130507103028.htm

Chapter Twenty-Five

307. Vasko, C. (n.d.). Foods that fight cancer. *Stand Up To Cancer.* Retrieved March 3, 2013, from http://www.standup2cancer.org/article_archive/view/foods_that_fight_cancer

308. Rock, C. L., Doyle, C., Demark–Wahnefried, W., Meyerhardt, J., Courneya, K. S., Schwartz, A. L., Bandera, E. V., Hamilton, K. K., Grant, B., McCullough, M., Byers, T., & Gansler, T. (2012). Nutrition and physical activity guidelines for cancer survivors. *CA: A Cancer Journal for Clinicians, 62,* 242-274.doi: 10.3322/caac.21142

309. Park, E. J., Lee, J. H., Yu, G.-Y., He, G., Ali, S. R., Holzer, R. G., Österreicher, C. H., Takahashi, H., & Karin, M. (2010). Dietary and genetic obesity promote liver inflammation and tumorigenesis by enhancing IL-6 and TNF expression. *Cell, 140*(2), 197–208. doi:10.1016/j.cell.2009.12.052

310. Obesity ups cancer risk, and here's how. (2010, January 21). *ScienceDaily.* Retrieved from http://www.sciencedaily.com /releases/2010/01/100121135713.htm

311. Park, E. J., Lee, J. H., Yu, G.-Y., He, G., Ali, S. R., Holzer, R. G., Österreicher, C. H., Takahashi, H., & Karin, M. (2010). Dietary and genetic obesity promote liver inflammation and tumorigenesis by enhancing IL-6 and TNF expression. *Cell, 140*(2), 197–208. doi:10.1016/j.cell.2009.12.052

312. Hsu, A., Wong, C. P., Yu, Z., Williams, D. E., Dashwood, R. H., & Ho, E. (2011). Promoter de-methylation of cyclin D2 by sulforaphane in prostate cancer cells. *Clinical Epigenetics, 3*(1), 3. doi:10.1186/1868-7083-3-3

313. Wolk, A., Larsson, S. C., Johansson, J.-E., & Ekman, P. (2006). Long-term fatty fish consumption and renal cell carcinoma incidence in women. *Journal of the American Medical Association, 296*(11), 1371–1376. doi:10.1001/jama.296.11.1371

314. Vasko, C. (n.d.). Foods that fight cancer. *Stand Up to Cancer.* Retrieved March 3, 2013, from http://www.standup2cancer.org/article_archive/view/foods_that_fight_cancer

315. Li, W. (2010, May). TED Talk: Can we eat to starve cancer? [Video file]. Retrieved from http://www.ted.com/talks/william_li.html

316. Haykowsky, M., Scott, J., Esch, B., Schopflocher, D., Myers, J., Paterson, I., Warburton, D., Jones, L., & Clark, A. M. (2011). A meta-analysis of the effects of exercise training on left ventricular remodeling following myocardial infarction: Start early and go longer for greatest exercise benefits on remodeling. *Trials, 12*(1), 92. doi:10.1186/1745-6215-12-92

317. Heart needs work after heart attack: New study challenges the notion that the heart must rest. *ScienceDaily.* (2011, April 14). Retrieved April 19, 2012, from http://www.sciencedaily.com /releases/2011/04/110414131845.htm

318. Trivedi, M. H., Greer, T. L., Church, T. S., Carmody, T. J., Grannemann, B. D., Galper, D. I., Dunn, A. L., Earnest, C. P., Sunderajan, P., Henley, S. S., & Blair, S. N. (2011). Exercise as an augmentation treatment for nonremitted major depressive disorder. *Journal of Clinical Psychiatry, 72*(05), 677–684. doi:10.4088/JCP.10m06743

319. Varkey, E., Cider, Å., Carlsson, J., & Linde, M. (2011). Exercise as migraine prophylaxis: A randomized study using relaxation and topiramate as controls. *Cephalalgia, 31*(14), 1428–1438. doi:10.1177/0333102411419681

320. Fitness reduces inflammation, study suggests. (2007, July 6). *ScienceDaily*. Retrieved April 19, 2012, from http://www.sciencedaily.com/releases/2007/07/070706115120. htm

321. Barrès, R., Yan, J., Egan, B., Treebak, J. T., Rasmussen, M., Fritz, T., Caidahl, K., Krook, A., O'Gorman, D. J., & Zierath, J. R. (2012). Acute exercise remodels promoter methylation in human skeletal muscle. *Cell Metabolism, 15*(3), 405–411. doi:10.1016/j. cmet.2012.01.001

322. Yusuf, S., Hawken, S., Ounpuu, S., Dans, T., Avezum, A., Lanas, F., McQueen, M., Budaj, A., Pais, P., Varigos, J., Lisheng, L., & INTERHEART Study Investigators (2004). Effect of potentially modifiable risk factors associated with myocardial infarction in 52 countries (the INTERHEART study): Case-control study. *Lancet, 364*(9438), 937–952. doi:10.1016/S0140-6736(04)17018-9

323. Women's Heart Foundation. (n.d.). Women and heart disease. [Fact sheet]. Retrieved June 5, 2013 from http://www.womensheart.org/content/heartdisease/heart_disease_facts.asp

324. Winslow, R. (2012, April 16). The guide to beating a heart attack: First line of defense is lowering risk, even when genetics isn't on your side. *Wall Street Journal*. Retrieved from http://online.wsj.com/article/SB10001424052702304818404577347982400815676.html

325. Belalcazar, L. M., Lang, W., Haffner, S. M., Hoogeveen, R. C., Pi-Sunyer, F. X. Schwenke, D. C., Balasubramanyam, A., Tracy, A. P., Kriska, A. P., Ballantyne, C. M., & Look AHEAD Research Group. (2012). Adiponectin and the mediation of HDL cholesterol change with improved lifestyle: The Look AHEAD Study. *Journal of Lipid Research, 53*(12), 2726-2733. doi: 10.1194/jlr.M030213

Chapter Twenty-Six

326. Knäuper, B., McCollam, A., Rosen-Brown, A., Lacaille, J., Kelso, E., & Roseman, M. (2011). Fruitful plans: Adding targeted mental imagery to implementation intentions increases fruit consumption. *Psychology & Health, 26*(5), 601–617. doi:10.1080/08870441003703218

327. Read, D., & van Leeuwen, B. (1998). Predicting hunger: The effects of appetite and delay on choice. *Organizational Behavior and Human Decision Processes, 76*(2), 189–205. doi:10.1006/obhd.1998.2803

328. Reynolds, G. (2012, February 1). Exercise as housecleaning for the body. *New York Times: Well*. [Web log]. Retrieved from http://well.blogs.nytimes.com/2012/02/01/exercise-as-housecleaning-for-the-body/

329. He, C., Bassik, M. C., Moresi, V., Sun, K., Wei, Y., Zou, Z., An, Z., Loh, J., Fisher, J., Sun, Q., Korsmeyer, S., Packer, M., May, H. I., Hill, J. A., Virgin, H. W., Gilpin, C., Xiao G., Bassel-Duby, R., Scherer, P. E., & Levine, B. (2012). Exercise-induced BCL2-regulated autophagy is required for muscle glucose homeostasis. *Nature, 481*, 511-515. doi:10.1038/nature10758

330. Reynolds, G. (2012, November 7). Can exercise protect the brain from fatty foods? *New York Times: Well*. [Web log]. Retrieved from http://well.blogs.nytimes.com/2012/11/07/can-exercise-protect-the-brain-from-fatty-foods/

331. Martin, D. (2011). Physical activity benefits and risks on the gastrointestinal system. *Southern Medical Journal, 104*(12), 831–837. doi:10.1097/SMJ.0b013e318236c263

332. Pace–Schott, E. F., Nave, G., Morgan, A., Spencer, R. M. C., (2012). Sleep–dependent modulation of affectively guided decision–making. *Journal of Sleep Research, 21*(1), 30–39. doi:10.1111/j.1365-2869.2011.00921.x.

333. Sio, U. N., Monaghan, P., & Ormerod, T. (2013). Sleep on it, but only if it is difficult: Effects of sleep on problem solving. *Memory & Cognition, 41*(2): 159-166. doi: 10.3758/s13421-012-0256-7

Chapter Twenty-Seven

334. Boutelle, K. N., Cafri, G., & Crow, S. J. (2012). Parent predictors of child weight. Change in family based behavioral obesity treatment. *Obesity, 20*(7), 1539-1543. doi:10.1038/oby.2012.48

335. Families that eat together may be the healthiest, new evidence confirms. (2012, April 23). *ScienceDaily.* Retrieved from http://www.sciencedaily.com/releases/2012/04/120423184157.htm

336. Eating berries may activate the brain's natural housekeeper for healthy aging. (2010, August 23).*ScienceDaily.* Retrieved from http://www.sciencedaily.com /releases/2010/08/100823142927.htm

337. Tulipani, S., Alvarez-Suarez, J. M., Busco, F., Bompadre, S., Quiles, J. L., Mezzetti, B., & Battino, M. (2011). Strawberry consumption improves plasma antioxidant status and erythrocyte resistance to oxidative haemolysis in humans. *Food Chemistry, 128*(1), 180–186. doi:10.1016/j.foodchem.2011.03.025

338. Maher, P., Dargusch, R., Ehren, J. L., Okada, S., Sharma, K., & Schubert, D. (2011). Fisetin lowers methylglyoxal dependent protein glycation and limits the complications of diabetes. *PLoS ONE, 6*(6), e21226. doi:10.1371/journal.pone.0021226

339. Eating berries may lower risk of Parkinson's. (2011, February 17). *ScienceDaily.* Retrieved April 18, 2012, from http://www.sciencedaily.com /releases/2011/02/110213162726.htm

340. Miller, M. G., & Shukitt-Hale, B. (2012). Berry fruit enhances beneficial signaling in the brain. *Journal of Agricultural and Food Chemistry, 60(23),* 5709-5715. doi:10.1021/jf2036033

341. Devore, E. E., Kang, J. H., Breteler, M. M. B., & Grodstein, F. (2012). Dietary intakes of berries and flavonoids in relation to cognitive decline. *Annals of Neurology, 72*(1), 135-143. doi:10.1002/ana.23594

342. Dunn, E., & Norton, M. (2012, July 7). Don't indulge. Be happy. *The New York Times.* Retrieved from http://www.nytimes.com/2012/07/08/opinion/sunday/dont-indulge-be-happy.htm

343. Ried, K., Sullivan, T., Fakler, P., Frank, O. R., & Stocks, N. P. (2010). Does chocolate reduce blood pressure? A meta-analysis. *BMC Medicine, 8*(1), 39. doi:10.1186/1741-7015-8-39

344. Yasuda, A., Natsume, M., Osakabe, N., Kawahata, K., & Koga, J. (2011). Cacao polyphenols influence the regulation of apolipoprotein in HepG2 and Caco2 cells. *Journal of Agriculture and Food Chemistry, 59*(4), 1470–1476. doi:10.1021/jf103820b

345. Buijsse, B., Weikert, C., Drogan, D., Bergmann, M., & Boeing, H. (2010). Chocolate consumption in relation to blood pressure and risk of cardiovascular disease in German adults. *European Heart Journal, 31*(13), 1616–1623. doi:10.1093/eurheartj/ehq068

346. Crum, A. J., & Langer, E. J. (2007). Mind-set matters: Exercise and the placebo effect. *Psychological Science, 18*(2), 165–171. doi:10.1111/j.1467-9280.2007.01867.x

347. Mcguire, K. A. & Ross, R. (2011). Incidental physical activity is positively associated with cardiorespiratory fitness. *Medicine & Science in Sports & Exercise, 43*(11), 2189–2194. doi:10.1249/MSS.0b013e31821e4ff2

Chapter Twenty-Eight

348. Hsu, A., Wong, C. P., Yu, Z., Williams, D. E., Dashwood, R. H., & Ho, E. (2011). Promoter de-methylation of cyclin D2 by sulforaphane in prostate cancer cells. *Clinical Epigenetics, 3*(1), 3. doi:10.1186/1868-7083-3-3

349. Clarke, J. D., Hsu, A., Yu, Z., Dashwood, R. H., & Ho, E. (2011). Differential effects of sulforaphane on histone deacetylases, cell cycle arrest and apoptosis in normal prostate cells versus hyperplastic and cancerous prostate cells. *Molecular Nutrition & Food Research, 55*(7), 999–1009. doi:10.1002/mnfr.201000547

350. From and for the heart, my dear valentine: Broccoli. (2008, January 21). *ScienceDaily*. Retrieved from http://www.sciencedaily.com /releases/2008/01/080121091349.htm

351. Eating cruciferous vegetables may improve breast cancer survival. (2012, April 3). *ScienceDaily*. Retrieved from http://www.sciencedaily.com /releases/2012/04/120403153531.htm

352. Eating broccoli could guard against arthritis. (2010, September 15). *ScienceDaily*. Retrieved from http://www.sciencedaily.com /releases/2010/09/100915084504.htm

353. Broccoli may help protect against respiratory conditions like asthma. (2009, March 2). *ScienceDaily*. Retrieved from http://www.sciencedaily.com /releases/2009/03/090302133218.htm

354. Farnham, M. W., & Kopsell, D. A. (2009). Importance of genotype on carotenoid and chlorophyll levels in broccoli heads. *HortScience, 44*(5), 1248–1253.

355. Li, Y., Innocentin, S., Withers, D. R., Roberts, N. A., Gallagher, A. R., Grigorieva, E. F., Wilhelm, C., & Veldhoen, M. (2011). Exogenous stimuli maintain intraepithelial lymphocytes via aryl hydrocarbon receptor activation. *Cell, 147*(3), 629–640. doi:10.1016/j.cell.2011.09.025

356. Kliff, S. (2012, June 14). Americans actually really like broccoli. *The Washington Post: Wonkblog*. [Web log]. Retrieved from http://www.washingtonpost.com/blogs/ezra-klein/post/americans-actually-really-like-broccoli/2012/06/14/gJQAsMbOcV_blog.html

357. Ranjit, N., Evans, M. H., Byrd-Williams, C., Evans, A. E., & Hoelscher, D. M. (2010). Dietary and activity correlates of sugar-sweetened beverage consumption among adolescents. *Pediatrics, 126*(4), e754–e761. doi:10.1542/peds.2010-1229

358. Stein, J. (2011, August 31). Half of all Americans drink a sugary beverage daily. *Los Angeles Times*. Retrieved from http://articles.latimes.com/2011/aug/31/news/la-heb-sugary-beverages-cdc-20110831

359. Malik, V. S., Popkin, B. M., Bray, G. A., Després, J.-P., Willett, W. C., & Hu, F. B. (2010). Sugar-sweetened beverages and risk of metabolic syndrome and type 2 diabetes: A meta-analysis. *Diabetes Care, 33*(11), 2477–2483. doi:10.2337/dc10-1079

360. Mueller, N. T., Odegaard, A., Anderson, K., Yuan, J.-M., Gross, M., Koh, W.-P., & Pereira, M. A. (2010). Soft drink and juice consumption and risk of pancreatic cancer: The Singapore Chinese Health Study. *Cancer Epidemiology Biomarkers & Prevention, 19*(2), 447–455. doi:10.1158/1055-9965.EPI-09-0862

361. Neale, T. (2012, March 12). Sugary drinks tied to more heart attacks. *MedPage Today*. Retrieved from http://www.medpagetoday.com/Cardiology/MyocardialInfarction/31614

362. de Koning, L., Malik, V. S., Kellogg, M. D., Rimm, E. B., Willett, W. C., & Hu, F. B. (2012). Sweetened beverage consumption, incident coronary heart disease and biomarkers of risk in men. *Circulation, 125*(14), *1735-1741*. doi:10.1161/CIRCULATIONAHA.111.067017

363. Wade, L. (2013, March 19). Sugary drinks linked to 180,000 deaths worldwide. *CNN Health*. Retrieved from http://www.cnn.com/2013/03/19/health/sugary-drinks-deaths/index.html

364. Diet soda may raise odds of vascular events; Salt linked to stroke risk. (2011, February 9). *ScienceDaily*. Retrieved from http://www.sciencedaily.com /releases/2011/02/110209121653.htm

365. Hold the diet soda? Sweetened drinks linked to depression, coffee tied to lower risk. (2013, January 8). *ScienceDaily*. Retrieved from http://www.sciencedaily.com /releases/2013/01/130108162135.htm

366. Gardener, H., Rundek, T., Markert, M., Wright, C., Elkind, M., & Sacco, R. (2012). Diet soft drink consumption is associated with an increased risk of vascular events in the Northern Manhattan study. *Journal of General Internal Medicine, 27*(9), 1120-1126. doi:10.1007/s11606-011-1968-2

367. Sengpiel, V., Elind, E., Bacelis, J., Nilsson, S., Grove, J., Myhre, R., Haugen, M., Meltzer, H. M., Alexander, J., Jacobsson, B., & Brantsæter, A. (2013). Maternal caffeine intake during pregnancy is associated with birth weight but not with gestational length: results from a large prospective observational cohort study. *BMC Medicine, 11,* 42. doi: 10.1186/1741-7015-11-42

368. Lucas, M., Mirzaei, F., Pan, A., Okereke, O. I., Willett, W. C., O'Reilly, E. J., Koenen, K., et al. (2011). Coffee, caffeine, and risk of depression among women. *Archives of Internal Medicine, 171*(17), 1571–1578. doi:10.1001/archinternmed.2011.393

369. Kawachi, I., Willett, W. C., Colditz, G. A., Stampfer, M. J., & Speizer, F. E. (1996). A prospective study of coffee drinking and suicide in women. *Archives of Internal Medicine, 156*(5), 521–525. doi:10.1001/archinte.1996.00440050067008

370. Galeone, C., Tavani, A., Pelucchi, C., Turati, F., Winn, D. M., Levi, F., Yu, G. P., Morgenstern, H., Kelsey, K., Dal Maso, L., Purdue, M. P., McClean, M., Talamini, R., Hayes, R. B., Franceshi, S., Schantz, S., Zhang, Z. F., Ferro, G., Chuang, S. C., Boffetta, P., La Vecchia, C., & Hasibe, M. (2010). Coffee and tea intake and risk of head and neck cancer: Pooled analysis in the International Head and Neck Cancer Epidemiology Consortium. *Cancer Epidemiology Biomarkers & Prevention, 19*(7), 1723–1736. doi:10.1158/1055-9965.EPI-10-0191

371. Freedman, N. D., Park, Y., Abnet, C. C., Hollenbeck, A. R., & Sinha, R. (2012). Association of coffee drinking with total and cause-specific mortality. *New England Journal of Medicine, 366*(20), 1891–1904. doi:10.1056/NEJMoa1112010

372. Ascherio, A., Weisskopf, M. G., O'Reilly, E. J., McCullough, M. L., Calle, E. E., Rodriguez, C., & Thun, M. J. (2004). Coffee consumption, gender, and Parkinson's disease mortality in the cancer prevention study II cohort: The modifying effects of estrogen. *American Journal of Epidemiology, 160*(10), 977–984. doi:10.1093/aje/kwh312

373. Graham, T. E., Hibbert, E., & Sathasivam, P. (1998). Metabolic and exercise endurance effects of coffee and caffeine ingestion. *Journal of Applied Physiology, 85*(3), 883–889.

374. Why coffee protects against diabetes. (2011, January 13). *ScienceDaily.* Retrieved from http://www.sciencedaily.com /releases/2011/01/110113102200.htm

375. Exercise and caffeine change your DNA in the same way, study suggests. (2012, March 6). *ScienceDaily.* Retrieved from http://www.sciencedaily.com/releases/2012/03/120306131254.htm

376. Barrès, R., Yan, J., Egan, B., Treebak, J. T., Rasmussen, M., Fritz, T., Caidahl, K., Krook, A., O'Gorman, D. J., Zierath, J. R. (2012). Acute exercise remodels promoter methylation in human skeletal muscle. *Cell Metabolism, 15*(3), 405–411. doi:10.1016/j.cmet.2012.01.001

377. Tight ties, killer heels: Clothes make the fashion victims. (2012, February 21). *Wall Street Journal.* Retrieved from http://online.wsj.com/article/SB10001424052970204909104577235313412770808.html

378. Wong, V. (2012, March 7). Why Richard Branson won't wear a tie. *Bloomberg Businessweek.* Retrieved from http://www.businessweek.com/articles/2012-03-07/why-richard-branson-wont-wear-a-tie

Chapter Twenty-Nine

379. Lonser, R. R., Glenn, G. M., Walther, M., Chew, E. Y., Libutti, S. K., Linehan, W. M., & Oldfield, E. H. (2003). von Hippel-Lindau disease. *The Lancet, 361*(9374), 2059–2067. doi:10.1016/S0140-6736(03)13643-4

380. Wolk, A., Larsson, S. C., Johansson, J. E., & Ekman, P. (2006). Long-term fatty fish consumption and renal cell carcinoma incidence in women. *Journal of the American Medical Association, 296*(11), 1371–1376. doi:10.1001/jama.296.11.1371

381. McGuire, B. B. & Fitzpatrick, J. M. (2011). BMI and the risk of renal cell carcinoma. *Current Opinion in Urology, 21*(5), 356–361. doi:10.1097/MOU.0b013e32834962d5

382. Obesity, depression found to be root causes of daytime sleepiness. (2012, June 13). *ScienceDaily*. Retrieved from http://www.sciencedaily.com /releases/2012/ 06/120613091037.htm

383. Knutson, K. L. (2012). Does inadequate sleep play a role in vulnerability to obesity? *American Journal of Human Biology, 24*(3), 361–371. doi:10.1002/ajhb.22219

384. Losing weight, especially in the belly, improves sleep quality. (2012, November 6). *ScienceDaily*. Retrieved from http://www.sciencedaily.com/releases/2012/11/ 121106125450.htm

385. Sivak, M. (2006). Sleeping more as a way to lose weight. *Obesity Reviews, 7*(3), 295–296. doi:10.1111/j.1467-789X.2006.00262.x

386. Schwartz, T. (2011, March 3). Sleep is more important than food. *Harvard Business Review Blog Network*. [Web log]. Retrieved from http://blogs.hbr.org/schwartz/2011/03/ sleep-is-more-important-than-f.html

387. Jones, M. (2011, April 15). How little sleep can you get away with? *The New York Times*. Retrieved from http://www.nytimes.com/2011/04/17/magazine/mag-17Sleep-t. html

Chapter Thirty

388. Cantin, J., Lacroix, S., Tardif, J., & Nigam, A. (2012). 390 Does the adherence to a Mediterranean diet influence baseline and postprandial endothelial function? *Canadian Journal of Cardiology, 28*(5, Supplement), S245. doi:10.1016/j.cjca.2012.07.367

389. Williams, P. T., & Thompson, P. D. (2013). Walking versus running for hypertension, cholesterol, and diabetes mellitus risk reduction. *Arteriosclerosis, Thrombosis, and Vascular Biology, 33*(5), 1085–1091. doi:10.1161/ATVBAHA.112.300878

390. Wen, C. P., Wai, J. P. M., Tsai, M. K., Yang, Y. C., Cheng, T. Y. D., Lee, M.-C., Chan, H. T., Tsao, C. K., Tsai, S. P., & Wu, X. (2011). Minimum amount of physical activity for reduced mortality and extended life expectancy: A prospective cohort study. *The Lancet, 378*(9798), 1244–1253. doi:10.1016/S0140-6736(11)60749-6

391. Lee, I.-M., Djoussé, L., Sesso, H. D., Wang, L., & Buring, J. E. (2010). Physical activity and weight gain prevention. *Journal of the American Medical Association, 303*(12), 1173–1179. doi:10.1001/jama.2010.312

392. Maher, J. P., Doerksen, S. E., Elavsky, S., Hyde, A. L., Pincus, A. L., Ram, N., & Conroy, D. E. (2013). A daily analysis of physical activity and satisfaction with life in emerging adults. *Health Psychology, 32*(6), 647-656. doi: 10.1037/a0030129

393. Martikainen, S., Pesonen, A.-K., Lahti, J., Heinonen, K., Feldt, K., Pyhälä, R., Tammelin, T., Kajantie, E., Eriksson, J. G., Strandberg, T. E., & Räikkönen, K. (2013). Higher levels of physical activity are associated with lower hypothalamic-pituitary-adrenocortical axis reactivity to psychosocial stress in children. *Journal of Clinical Endocrinology & Metabolism, 98*, E619-E627. doi:10.1210/jc.2012-3745

394. Spiegel, K., Leproult, R., L'Hermite-Balériaux, M., Copinschi, G., Penev, P. D., & Van Cauter, E. (2004). Leptin levels are dependent on sleep duration: Relationships with sympathovagal balance, carbohydrate regulation, cortisol, and thyrotropin. *Journal of Clinical Endocrinology & Metabolism, 89*(11), 5762–5771. doi:10.1210/ jc.2004-1003

395. Taheri, S., Lin, L., Austin, D., Young, T., & Mignot, E. (2004). Short sleep duration is associated with reduced leptin, elevated ghrelin, and increased body mass index. *PLoS Medicine, 1*(3). doi:10.1371/journal.pmed.0010062

396. The good life: Good sleepers have better quality of life and less depression. (2011, June 15). *ScienceDaily*. Retrieved from http://www.sciencedaily.com/ releases/2011/06/110614101120.htm

397. Susman, E. (2012, June 11). Sleepy people make bad food choices. *MedPage Today*. Retrieved from http://www.sciencedaily.com/releases/2011/06/110614101120.htm

398. Brody, J. E. (2011, May 30). A good night's sleep isn't a luxury; it's a necessity. *The New York Times*. Retrieved from http://www.nytimes.com/2011/05/31/health/31brody.html

399. Lack of sleep? Keep away from the buffet. (2013, February 20). *ScienceDaily*. Retrieved from http://www.sciencedaily.com /releases/2013/02/130220084701.htm

400. The good life: Good sleepers have better quality of life and less depression. (2011, June 15). *ScienceDaily*. Retrieved from http://www.sciencedaily.com/releases/2011/06/110614101120.htm

Concluding Thoughts

401. Boutelle, K. N., Cafri, G., & Crow, S. J. (2012). Parent predictors of child weight change in family based behavioral obesity treatment. *Obesity, 20*(7), 1539-1543. doi:10.1038/oby.2012.48

Addional Readings

402. Loureiro, M. L., Yen, S. T., Nayga, R. M. (2012). The effects of nutritional labels on obesity. *Agricultural Economics, 43*(3), 333-342. doi: 10.1111/j.1574-0862.2012.00586.x

403. Kaluza, J., Wolk, A., & Larsson, S. C. (2012). Red meat consumption and risk of stroke: A meta-analysis of prospective studies. *Stroke, 43*(10), 2556-2560. doi:10.1161/STROKEAHA.112.663286

404. McDougall, C. (2011). *Born to run: A hidden tribe, superathletes, and the greatest race the world has never seen*. New York: Vintage.

405. Cushioned heel running shoes may alter adolescent biomechanics, performance. (2013, March 19). *ScienceDaily*. Retrieved from http://www.sciencedaily.com/releases/2013/03/130319091420.htm

406. Land on your toes, save your knees. (2010, October 6). *ScienceDaily*. Retrieved from http://www.sciencedaily.com /releases/2010/08/100811093013.htm

407. Lieberman, D. E., Venkadesan, M., Werbel, W. A., Daoud, A. I., D'Andrea, S., Davis, I. S., Mang'eni, R. O., & Pitsiladis, Y. (2010). Foot strike patterns and collision forces in habitually barefoot versus shod runners. *Nature, 463*(7280), 531–535. doi:10.1038/nature08723

408. De Oliveira, C., Watt, R., & Hamer, M. (2010). Toothbrushing, inflammation, and risk of cardiovascular disease: Results from Scottish Health Survey. *BMJ, 340*, c2451–c2451. doi:10.1136/bmj.c2451

Acknowledgements

Nearly 10 years ago, one of my closest friends, publishing guru Dr. Piotr Juszkiewicz, encouraged me to write a book on this topic. He argued that my personal experiences and the research I had accumulated on health and wellness could benefit a wider audience. While I was not ready to work on this type of book at the time, his idea planted a seed that stuck with me over the years.

A year ago, after losing far too many friends and loved ones to preventable illnesses, I decided to step away from my job and dedicate *all* of my time to this book and to helping people to ultimately improve their health and well-being. At first, I was unsure about the best way to make this happen. Fortunately, Piotr agreed to publish *Eat Move Sleep* and join me in this mission, for which I am extraordinarily grateful.

In addition, this book and project would not have been possible without the overwhelming support of my friends and colleagues at Gallup. From the moment I explained *why* I was stepping away from my full-time role to work on this book, they provided encouragement and assistance at every turn. My colleagues also helped me figure out how to pursue this personal passion while still contributing to Gallup's big global mission.

One of the things I have learned about writing books over the years is that a draft gets better every time you share it with another person. So I share very early book drafts with hundreds of people and am grateful to *everyone* who reviewed rough drafts. Along the way, a handful of people see the potential for what the book can be and join me in reviewing multiple drafts and advising me on the overall project. A huge thanks to the following group for their extensive advice, time, and guidance: Geoff Brewer, Mary Cheddie, Jim Clifton, Jon Clifton, Dr. Maria de Guzman, Dr. Richard Edwards, Larry Emond, Dr. Steve Gladis, Dr. Jim Harter, Jennifer Hodges, Dr. Tim Hodges, Dr. Judy Krings, Allison Lowry, Tom Matson, Dr. Senia Maymin, Dr. Emily Meyer, Jan Miller, Jane Miller, Jason Milton, Andy Monnich, Tom Nolan, Steve O'Brien, Dr. Connie Rath, Doug Rath, Dr. Mary Reckmeyer, Keith Roberts, Linda Shostak, Dr. Jessica Tyler, and Trish Ward. And a very special thanks to my wife, Ashley, for reviewing every sentence, chapter, and title several times over.

ACKNOWLEDGEMENTS

When I first started work after college, I could not have imagined writing a single article for public consumption, let alone multiple books. That all changed when my mentor and grandfather, Don Clifton, said that he spotted some talent in my writing — which no one else had seen up to that point. Don also asked me to write a book with him during his final year of life, which went on to become *How Full Is Your Bucket?*

While working on that first book, Kelly Henry was the editor responsible for fixing a lot of sentences written by a guy who loved numbers and statistics ... but had never really learned how to write. Instead of just cleaning up my mess, she decided to teach me how to be a better writer at the sentence and paragraph level. It is hard to explain what a difference this approach has made. *Eat Move Sleep* is the seventh book I have worked on with Kelly, and I think she can see how her early investment in teaching (instead of just correcting) has paid off over time.

In launching this new book and publishing effort, one of the first things I realized is that our ability to reach more people is greatly dependent on the quality of the people and companies we identified as partners. The PGW and Perseus team led by Eric Kettunen, Susan Reich, Kevin Votel, and Kim Wylie have helped us ensure this book will be available far and wide. Our partners at Cave Henricks and Shelton Interactive, led by Barbara and Rusty, are working every day to shape and share the right ideas with others. Chin-Yee Lai worked with our team to design the book's jacket. Edward Bobel and Brent Wilcox helped us to ensure the book's layout made it easy to read.

Finally, on a personal note, I would like to thank the two people who cultivated my love of books and reading at a young age, my mother, Connie Rath, and grandmother, Shirley Clifton. Together they invested an extraordinary amount in my growth and development and continue to encourage and inspire me today. One of my favorite things to do nowadays is watch my wife Ashley, who built her career around helping kids learn to read, teach our two young children how to speak, read, and write. There is something miraculous about watching someone with a true gift in action. I have been fortunate enough over the years to be surrounded by extraordinarily talented and passionate people, for which I am eternally grateful.